The Book of
Irish Names

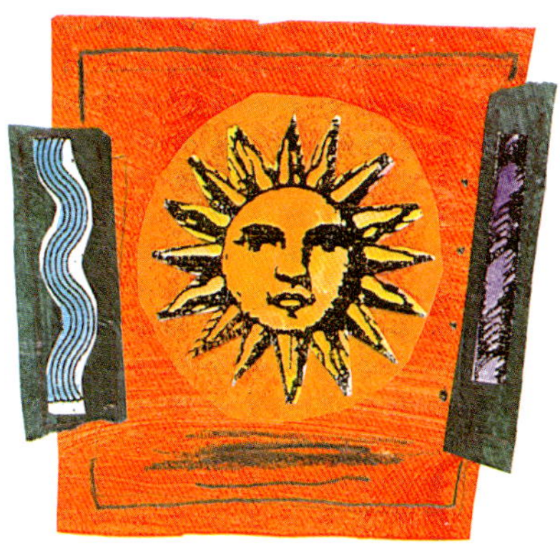

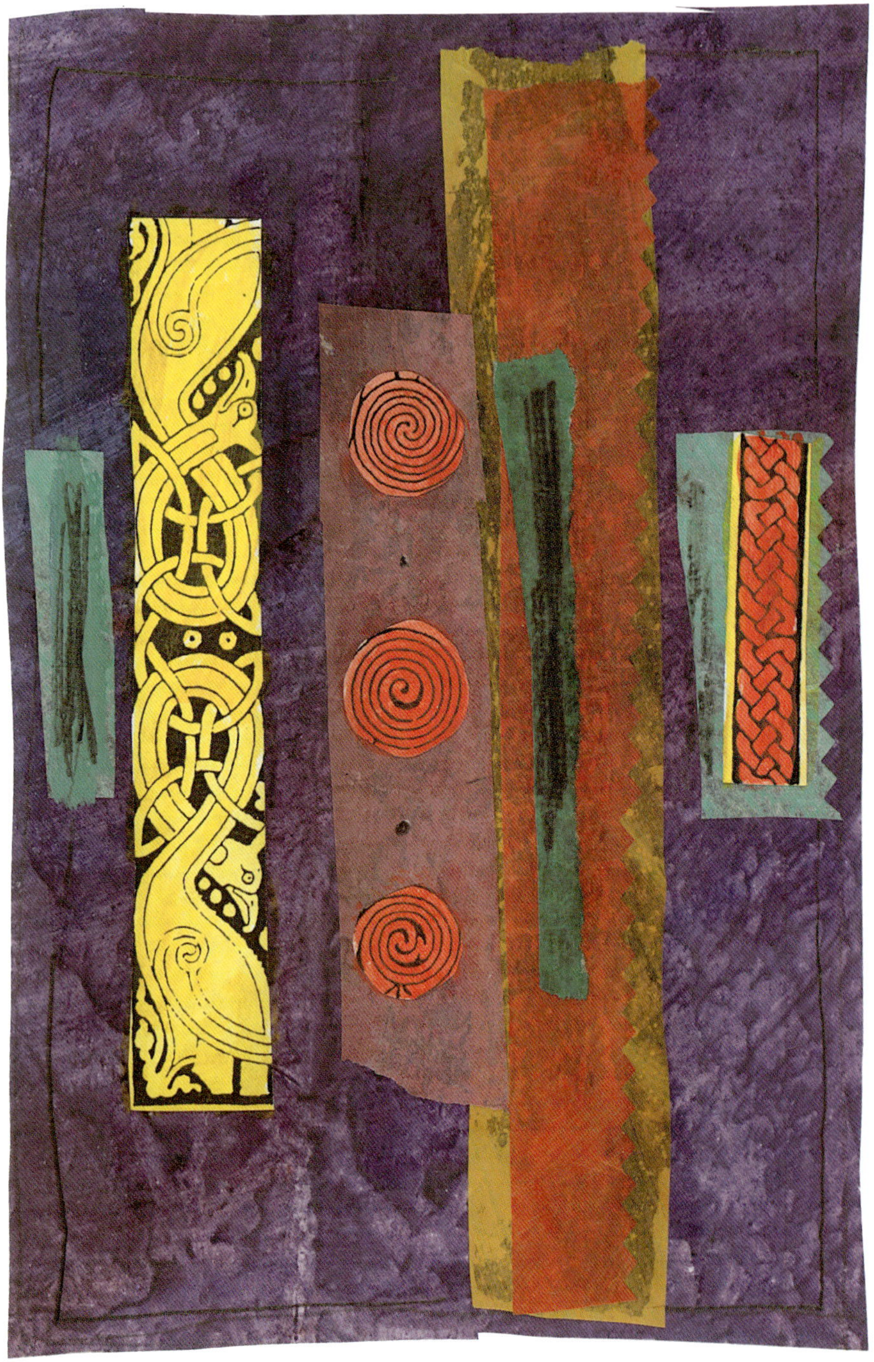

The Book of Irish Names

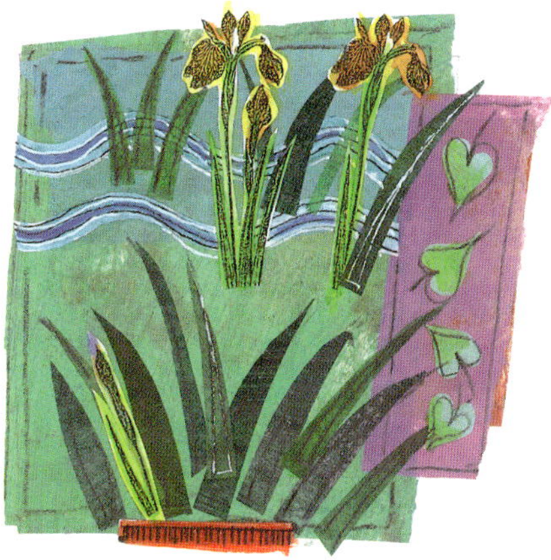

Iain Zaczek

Illustrated by
Jacqui Mair

Barnes & Noble Books
New York

This edition published by Barnes & Noble, Inc., by arrangement with Cico Books Ltd

2001 Barnes & Noble Books

M 10 9 8 7 6 5 4 3 2

ISBN 0-7607-2291-9

First published in Great Britain in 2000 by Cima Books

Designed by David Fordham

Illustrations by Jacqui Mair

Printed and bound in Singapore by Tien Wah Press

Contents

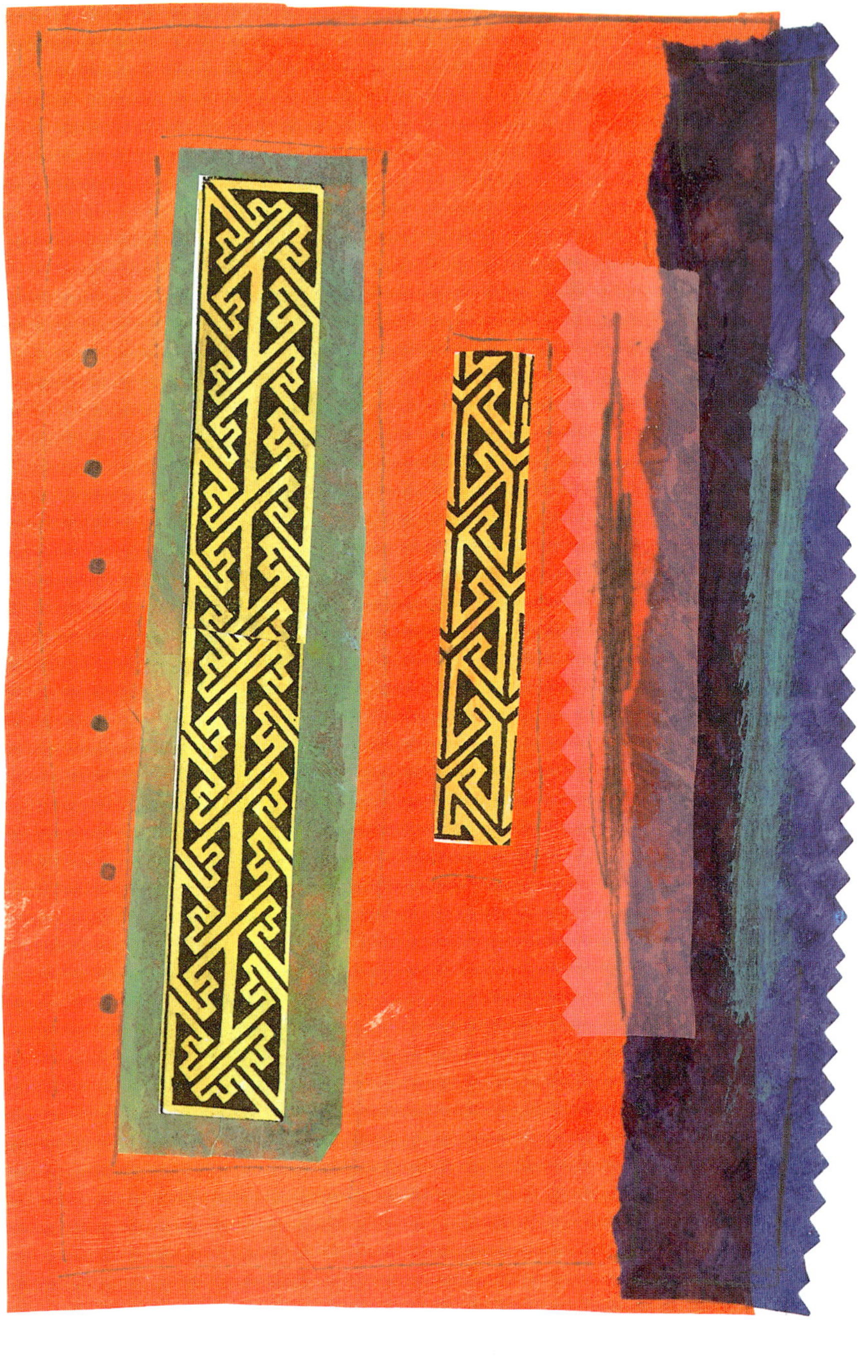

Introduction

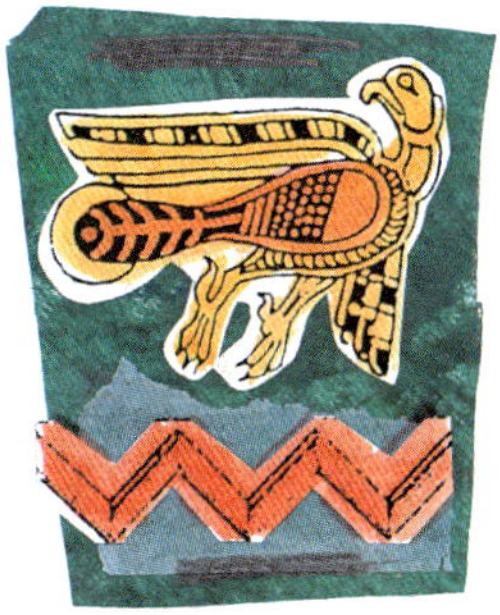

STEEPED IN THE HISTORY and romance of a rich cultural heritage, Irish names should provide a fruitful source of inspiration for any prospective parent. Whether they derive from ancient Celtic gods, native warrior-heroes, or pioneering saints, these names have now become popular throughout the Western world.

Ireland's early history was shaped by the Celts. Originating in central Europe, this ancient race migrated westwards, reaching Irish shores by around the 4th century BC. The Celts left an indelible mark on the culture of Scotland, Wales and Brittany, but it was in Ireland that they created their most lasting impact. Living beyond the frontiers of the Roman empire, the Irish were able to preserve the essentials of Celtic civilization for more than a thousand years. During this time, they produced such masterpieces as the Book of Kells, the Tara Brooch and the Celtic crosses at Clonmacnois.

Alone among the Celts, the Irish also kept alive a substantial body of ancient literature, giving a vivid account of their earliest gods and heroes. Most of these have been collected in two important story cycles – the Ulster cycle and the Fionn cycle. The Ulster cycle revolves around *The Cattle Raid of Cooley*, an epic tale in which Maeve, the Queen of Connaught, steals an enchanted bull. This leads her into conflict with the people of Ulster, led by their champion Cú Chulainn. The Fionn cycle, meanwhile, relates the exploits of Fionn mac Cumhaill and the warriors of the Fianna. They are in the service of the high king at Tara, and their adventures have often been likened to those of King Arthur and the knights of the Round Table.

Celtic culture survived in Ireland until the Middle Ages. It came under threat from the Viking raids, which began in the late 8th century, but remained a potent force until the coming of the Normans in the 12th century. Both of these foreign cultures have also made a contribution to the development of Irish names.

Boys' Names

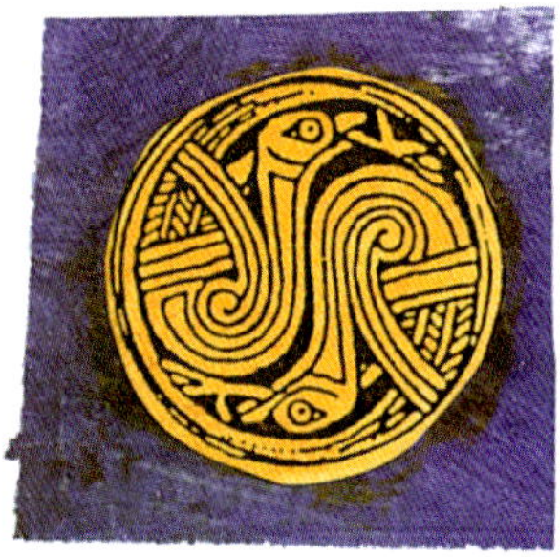

A high proportion of traditional boys' names have military or religious overtones, reflecting the two main preoccupations of early Irish society. Many are linked with the gods and warrior-heroes who featured in Ireland's ancient sagas. These include *The Cattle Raid of Cooley*, an epic tale of a war between Ulster and Connaught, and the colorful stories of the Fionn cycle, which recount the brave deeds of Fionn mac Cumhaill and the knights of the Fianna. Closely linked with these are the many names, which relate to animals or birds. In Irish legend, the ancient gods had the power to shape-shift into earthly creatures, and it is these deities who lie at the root of many 'animal' names.

The names of Irish saints have equally romantic associations. For their efforts in overturning the rule of the druids, they won great reverence and became the focus of a host of legends, which are every bit as enchanting as those normally reserved for fighting men.

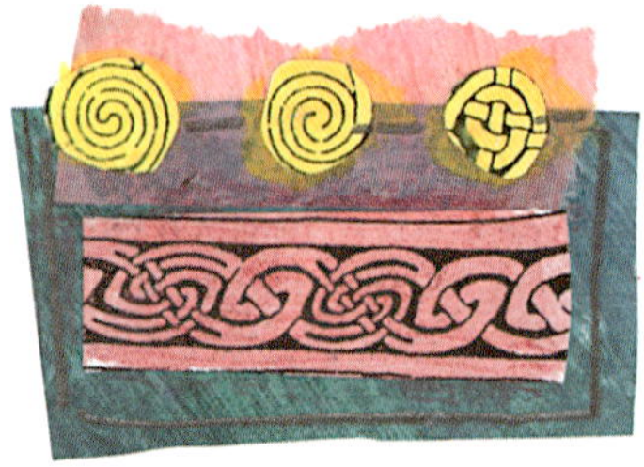

A

Adomnan

RELATED TO THE NAME of Adam, Adomnan (pronounced *A-dom-NAWN*) was highly popular in early Ireland. St. Adomnan (627–704) was born in Co. Donegal and later became abbot of Iona. He is most famous for his biography of St. Columba. In this, he described how the saint confronted a fearsome creature in Loch Ness – the first recorded mention of the Loch Ness monster.

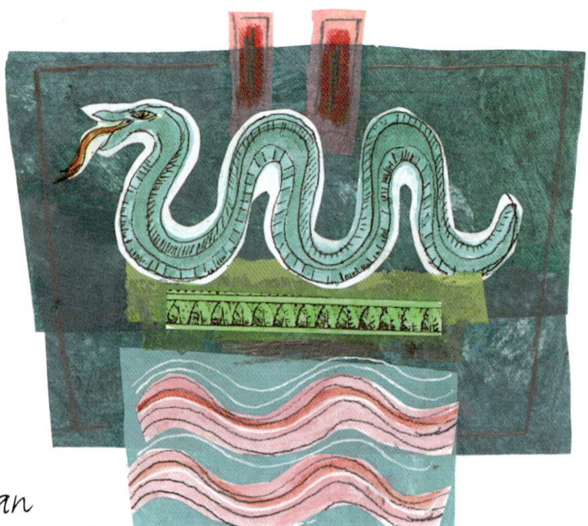

St Adomnan
(627–704)

Aidan

Aidan or Aedán means 'little fire', and has been a popular name in both Ireland and Scotland for many centuries. It is associated with many saints, most notably the missionary from Iona (c.600–51), who founded the monastery of Lindisfarne, and the Connaught monk, who built churches at Ferns, Co. Wexford, and Drumlane.

St Aidan, Iona (c.600–51)

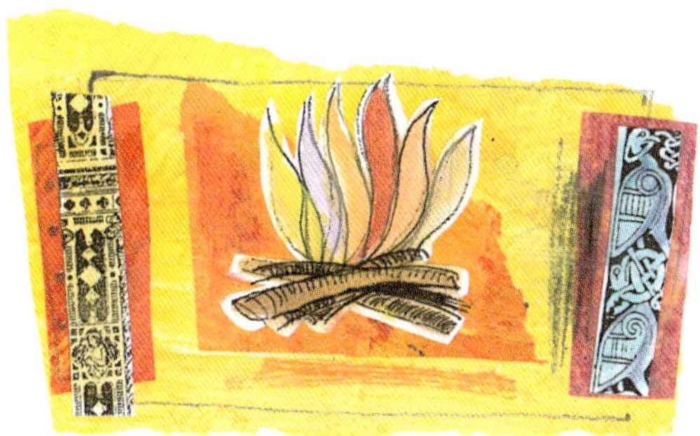

Ailill

Pronounced *A-lill*, this name is from a word meaning 'elf' or 'sprite'. This used to be one of the most popular names in Ireland. It has been linked with kings, saints and legendary heroes. The best-known of these was Ailill mac Máta, the consort of Queen Maeve in the ancient, epic tale of *The Cattle Raid of Cooley*.

Alan

This may derive from the Gaelic word for 'handsome' or 'cheerful', although a different Celtic origin has also been suggested. The Bretons (who were also Celts) developed the name Alain from their word for 'harmony' or 'peace'. Then, as a contingent in the Norman army, they brought it to both Britain and Ireland.

Aloysius

This name, pronounced *AL-LOO-ISH-US*, probably originated as a Latinized form of Louis. The name gained popularity in Catholic circles through the fame of Aloysius Gonzaga (1568–91), the Jesuit priest who was canonized for his work in a plague hospital. In Ireland, the name also provided a convenient translation for Lugaid, one of the most popular names in ancient times.

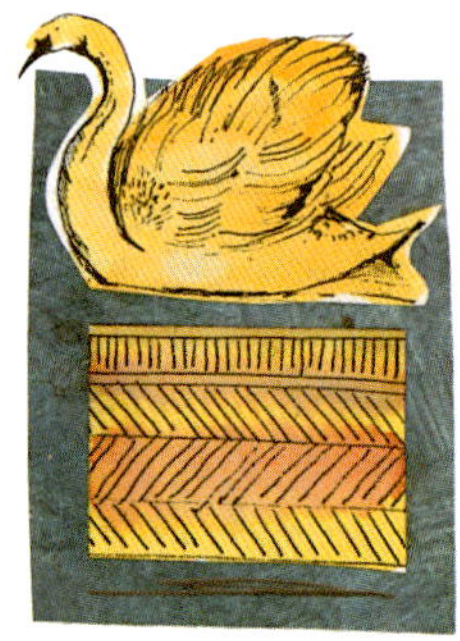

Angus, Aonghus

In its ancient form, Oenghus (pronounced *AYON-gus*), this was the Irish god of love. He dwelt in the fairy mound at Newgrange, which he won by stealth from his father. Oenghus rescued lovers in distress, though few romances were more troubled than his own. He had to turn himself into a swan to save his beloved from an enemy's spell.

Aodh

A modern form of Aed, an old Gaelic word for 'fire'. Many characters from Irish legend were named Aodh (pronounced *EY*, as in Hey), among them an ancient king from the northern territory of Airgialla. This warrior owned a shield called *Dubhghiolla* ('Dark Servant'), upon which the shape-shifting goddess of war used to perch, in the guise of a crow. The name can be anglicized as Hugh or Eugene.

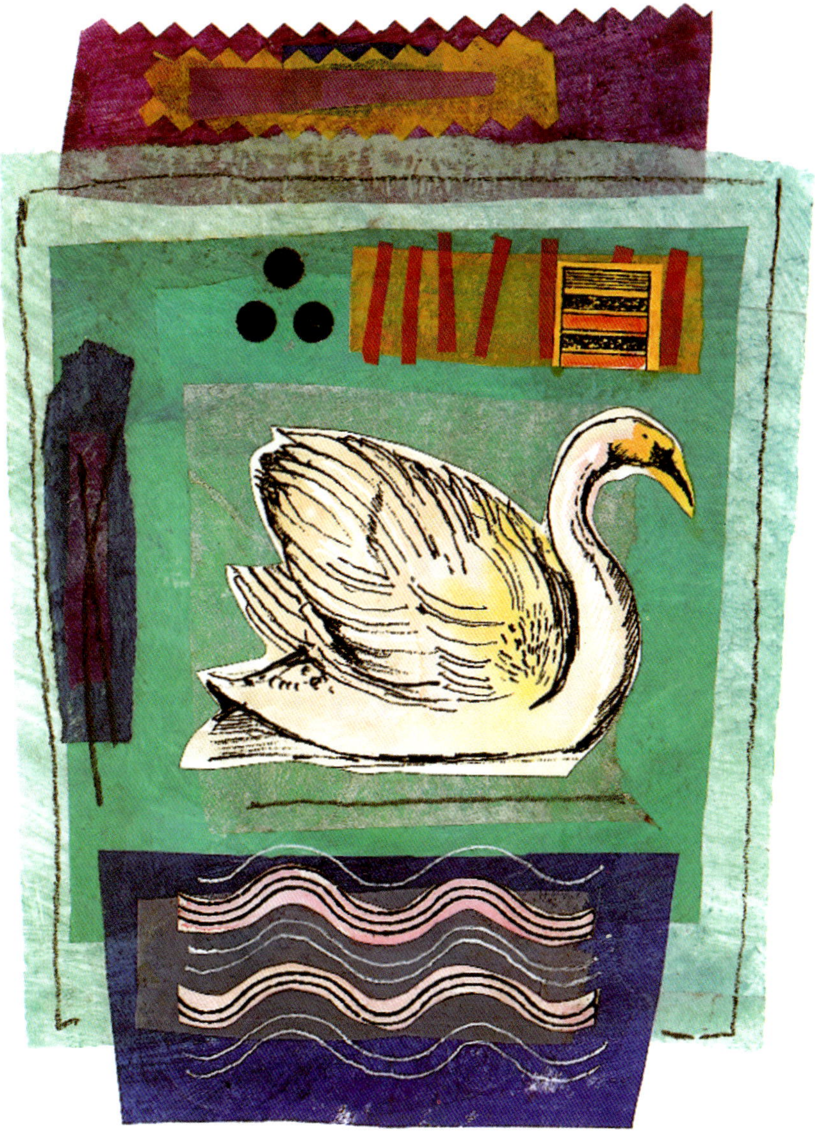

Oenghus, Irish god of love

ARDAL

IN COMMON WITH MANY traditional Irish names, Ardal was conceived in an ancient, warlike age, when martial qualities were much admired. It means 'highly courageous'. There may also be a linguistic link with Art or Arthur. The name has gained increasing prominence in recent years, popularized by such figures as the comedian and actor, Ardal O'Hanlon.

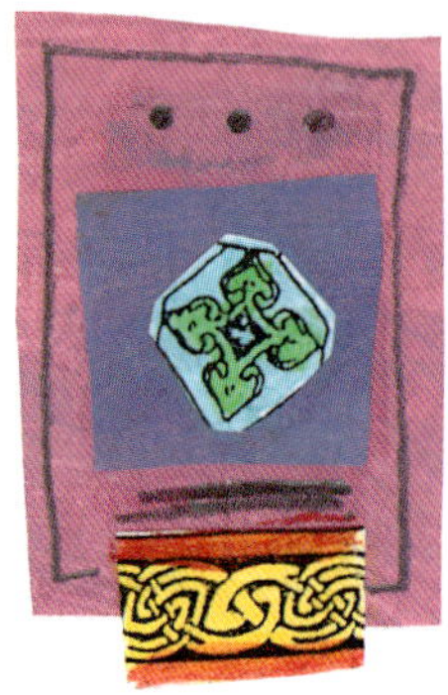

B

BEACAN, BEAGAN

PRONOUNCED *BEG-AWN*, this name comes from the Gaelic words for 'little one'. It was a favorite among the early Christian missionaries. One of these was the 6th-century Irish saint who founded the monastery of Westmeath. Another was Béccán mac Luigdech, a hermit on the island of Iona, who composed some of the oldest poetry in the Irish language.

BERCAN

THIS NAME COMES FROM the Gaelic words for 'little spear'. Despite its military overtones, it has mainly been associated with churchmen. There were no fewer than five Irish saints named Bercan, as well as a manuscript artist called Bercanus. Like Finbar, it is sometimes shortened to Barry.

Bran

Bran means 'raven', and is a popular name in all Celtic regions. It has been associated with poets, warriors and saints, but the best-known Irish example is the legendary hero, Bran mac Febail. He travelled to the magical Otherworld, enjoying its delights for many centuries. Finally becoming homesick, he returned to Ireland, where he crumbled into dust.

Bran mac Febail, legendary hero

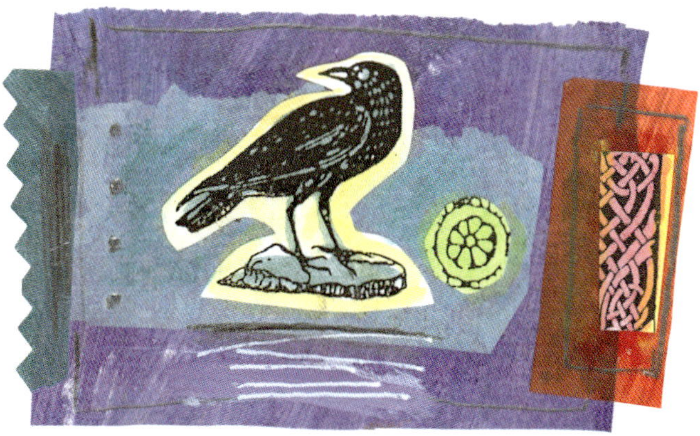

Branduff

Literally meaning 'black raven', this name was a favorite in early and medieval Ireland. Brandubh mac Echach was a 6th-century king of Leinster, who won resounding victories against his northern rivals. According to legend, he also tricked his rival, Mongán, into presenting him with his beautiful bride. Mongán spotted the ruse, however, and soon won her back.

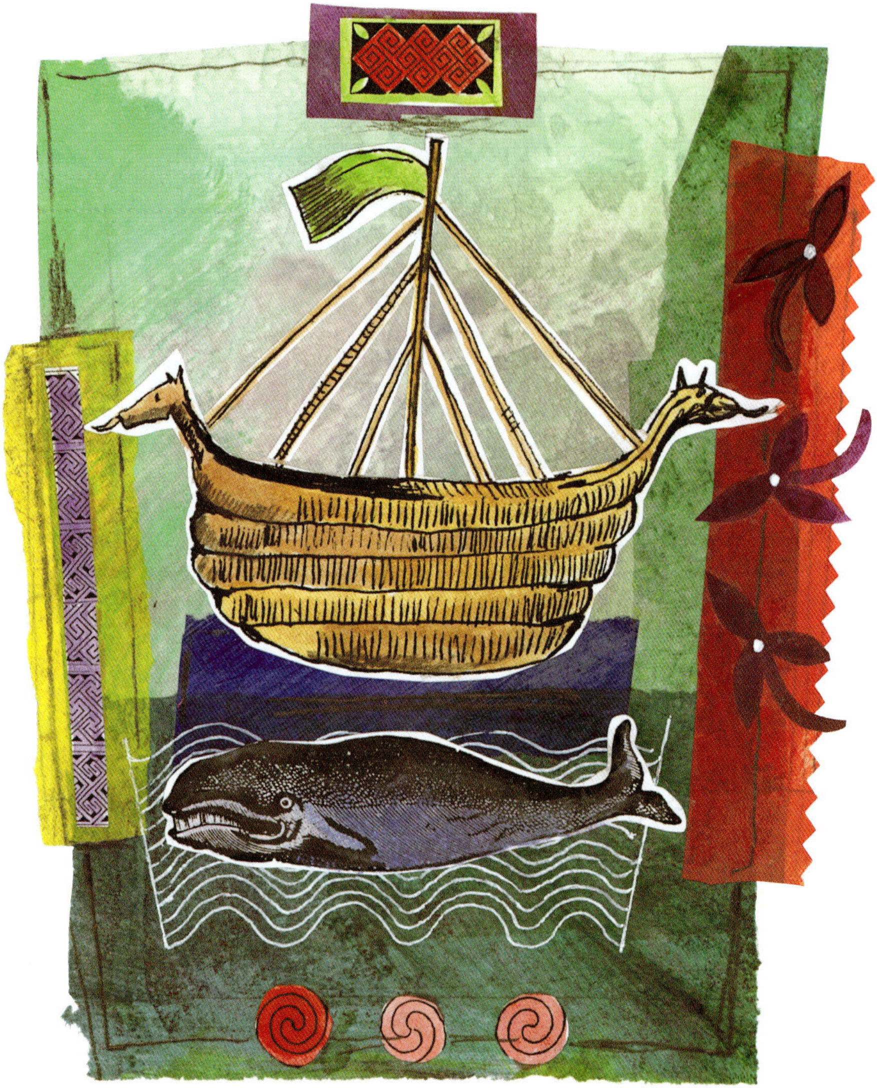

St Brendan the Navigator (c.486–c.575)

BRENDAN

DERIVING FROM *Bréanainn*, a Celtic word for 'prince', this name has been immortalized by two Irish saints. St. Brendan the Navigator (c.486–c.575) founded the monasteries of Clonfert (Co. Galway) and Ardfert (Co. Kerry), but is probably better known for the fabulous voyages which medieval chroniclers linked with his name. During these, it was said that he visited an island inhabited by birdmen, rode on the back of a whale, and landed on the shores of the Americas. Most of these expeditions were symbolic, spiritual journeys but in the 1970s several attempts were made to recreate his transatlantic voyages in a primitive curragh. An account of one of these ventures can be found in Tim Severin's *The Brendan Voyage* (1978).

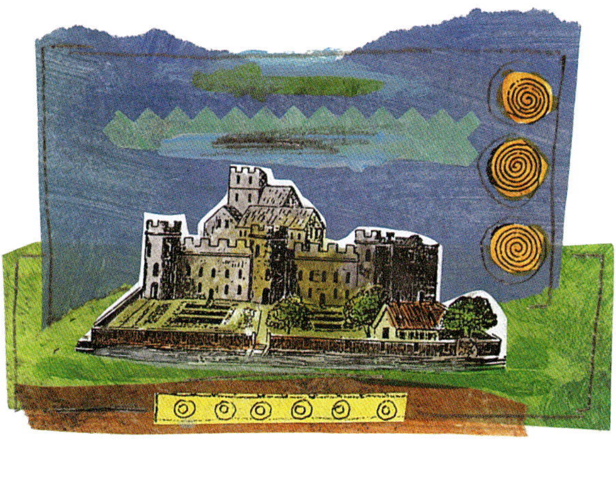

Brendan

By the standards of the time, the saint was well travelled. He is thought to have visited Scotland, travelled to Brittany with St. Malo, and become abbot of a Welsh monastery. His less famous compatriot was Brendan of Birr (d.573), a follower of St. Columba. In recent times the name has become associated with the playwright, Brendan Behan (1923–64), who wrote *The Quare Fellow* (1954) and *The Hostage* (1958).

Brian

The origin of this name is uncertain, although it may come from a Celtic word for 'high' or 'noble'. There was a minor deity in the Irish pantheon called Brian, but the name will always be most closely associated with Brian Boru, the greatest of Ireland's warrior-kings. He won the crucial Battle of Clontarf (1014), repelling an army of Danish invaders.

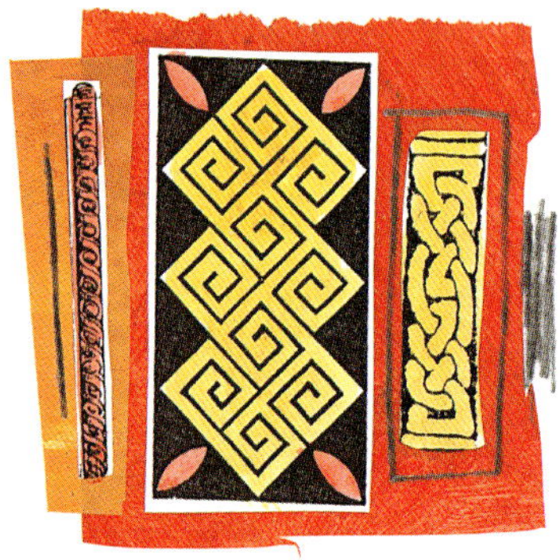

C

Cael

From an ancient word meaning 'slender', Cael (pronounced *KALE*) was a romantic hero of Irish legend. He courted Créd, the fairy daughter of King Cairbre of Kerry, wooing her with his poetic skills. Charmed by his verses, she agreed to become his bride and gave him a magic suit of armour as a token of her love.

Caffar

Caffar (pronounced *KAFF-AR*) and its variant, Cathbharr, both come from the Gaelic word for 'helmet'. In the past, it has also been used as a surname. In this context, it is most closely associated with the O'Donnells, who were the ruling dynasty in Tyrconnel, Co. Donegal, up until the 17th century.

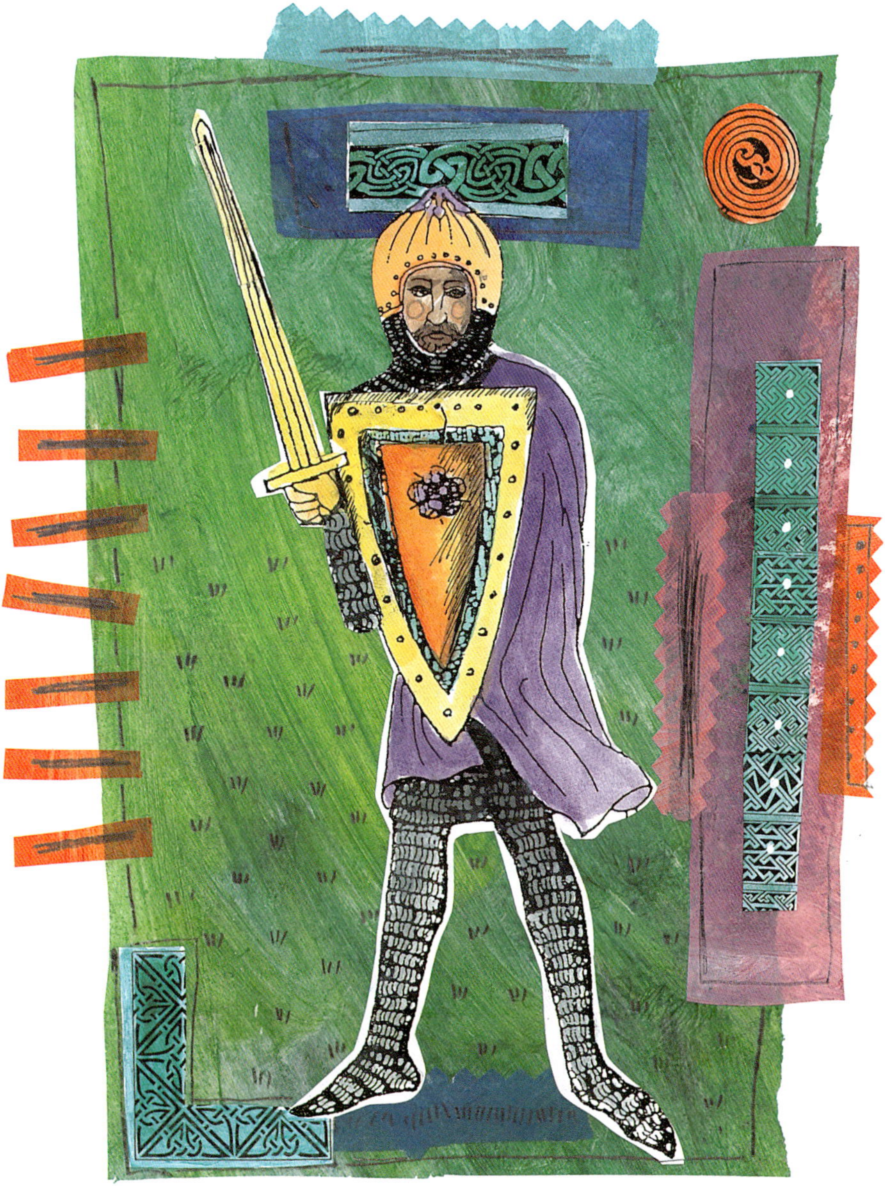

Brian Boru, 11th-century warrior-king

Cailitin, Calatin

Pronounced *KAL-I-TEEN*, this is an unusual name, which stems from a warrior-druid in *The Cattle Raid of Cooley*. Cailitin was an ally of Queen Maeve of Connaught and, on her behalf, he and his kinsmen did battle with Cú Chulainn, the champion of Ulster. In more recent times, the popularity of the name has been revived by W.B. Yeats, who used it for a character in *The Countess Cathleen* (1892).

Callaghan

Callaghan (pronounced *KALL-A-HAN*) is a diminutive of *ceallach*, meaning 'strife'. The name has been associated with a saint from Clontibret and a 10th-century king of Munster, but in modern times it has become more familiar as a surname. This trend is gradually being reversed in the US. Like Cathal, it is often shortened to Cal.

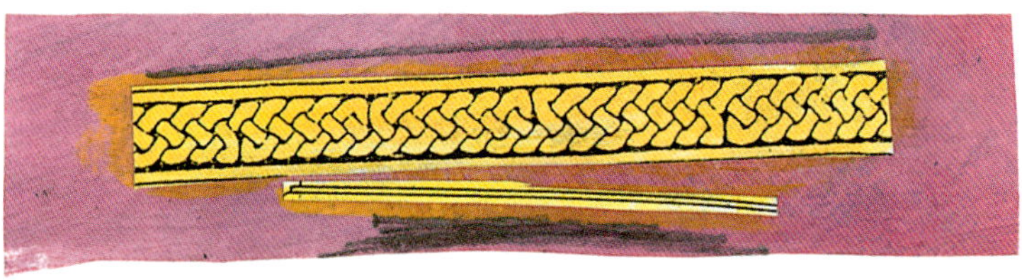

O Caiside family of Co. Fermanagh

Cassidy

Deriving from the Gaelic word for 'curly-haired', Cassidy first rose to prominence as a surname, associated with the O Caiside family of Co. Fermanagh – the hereditary physicians to the Maguire chieftains. In the US, it has become popular as a name for either boys or girls.

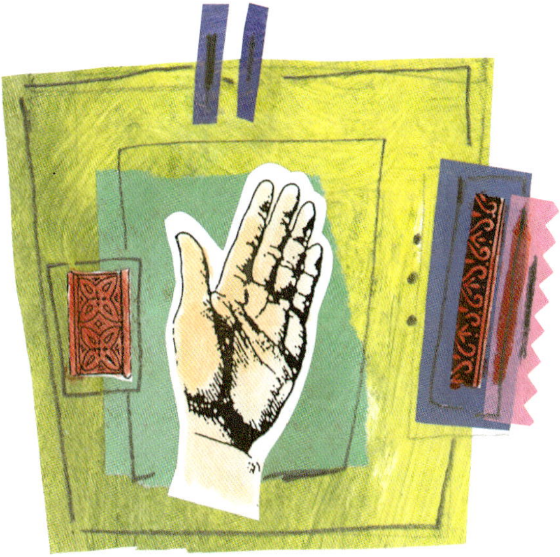

Cathal Crobderg,
13th-century prince

Cathal

Meaning 'strong in battle', this Gaelic name was extremely popular in medieval Ireland. It is linked with the 7th-century saint, who ran a monastic school at Lismore, and was also the name of a 13th-century prince, Cathal Crobderg ('of the red hand'). His nickname stemmed from a distinctive birthmark, which enabled him to prove his identity and secure the throne of Connaught.

Cathan

Stemming from the Irish word for 'battle' (*cath*), this is one of many names which dates back to an ancient time, when warlike qualities were much admired. As O Catháin ('the descendants of Cathan'), it became a popular family name in Galway and Ulster. It is frequently anglicized as Kane or Kean.

Cian

Meaning 'ancient', Cian (pronounced *KEE-an*) was a popular name for characters in early Irish mythology. Famously, Cian was the father of Lug, the sun-god. As an act of revenge he seduced the daughter of Balor, an evil king with a basilisk eye, after the latter had stolen his magic cow. As a result of this unhappy union, Lug was conceived.

Clancy

Deriving from the words for 'red' (*flann*) and 'battle' (*cath*), this signified a 'red-haired warrior'. The linguistic transformation stemmed from its use as a surname, Mac Fhlannchaidh ('son of the red-haired warrior'), most notably by a family of hereditary brehons (judges) in Co. Clare. In the US, it has become popular as a first name.

Colin, which means 'young hound'

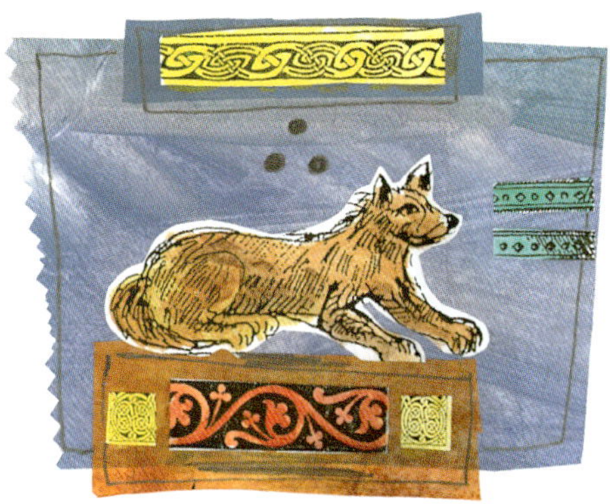

Colin

The probable source of this name is *coileán*, which means a 'young hound' or 'cub'. Alternatively, it may have developed as a pet form of Nicholas, which was popular in France and may have been brought across by the Normans. Its usage has increased enormously since the 18th century.

St Columba (c.521–97)

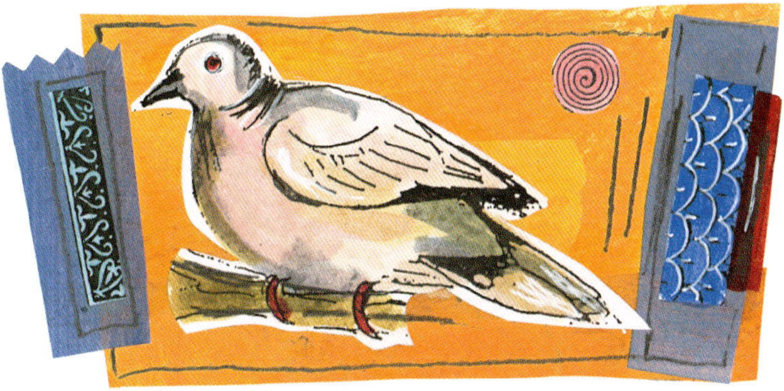

COLM

COLM IS THE GAELIC FORM of Columba, the Latin name for a 'dove'. As the traditional symbol of the Holy Ghost, it was an obvious choice for prospective churchmen. St. Columba (c.521–97) was born Colum-cille in Co. Donegal. He founded monasteries at Derry and Durrow, before setting off for Iona, to undertake the conversion of the Picts.

COLMAN

MEANING 'LITTLE DOVE', Colman came from the same root as Colm but developed into a separate name. Once again, it is strongly linked with the Church – Irish martyrologies list a staggering 300 saints with this name. The most celebrated are Colman of Cloyne (c.530–c.606), who worked initially as a royal bard, and Colman of Lindisfarne (d.676), who led the Irish delegation at the Synod of Whitby (664).

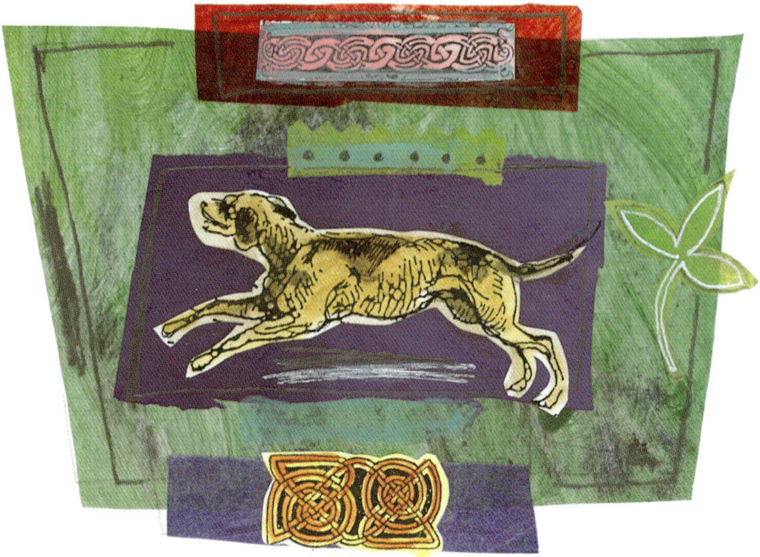

Conan the Barbarian

CONAN

MEANING 'LITTLE HOUND', Conan was the name of several legendary figures, as well as six Irish saints. More recently, it has been made famous by the creator of Sherlock Holmes, Sir Arthur Conan Doyle (1859–1930), who came from Irish stock, as well as the fictional adventures of Conan the Barbarian, which were written by Robert E. Howard (d.1936).

CONLEY

THE ORIGINS OF THIS traditional name are uncertain. Some believe that it comes from the Gaelic words for 'prudent fire'. Others argue that there is a link with St. Conleat (died c.520), the Irish monk who made liturgical vessels for St. Brigid, but was devoured by wolves while travelling to Rome.

Conn

Meaning 'wisdom' or 'reason', Conn was in widespread use in ancient Ireland. Dozens of legendary figures bear the name, the most celebrated of these being Conn Cétchathach (Conn of the Hundred Battles). He was an ancestor-deity, hailed as one of the first high kings of Ireland, and his descendants were the Connachta, who gave their name to the province of Connaught.

Conall, Connell

An old Celtic name, meaning 'mighty'. There was an Irish saint called Conall, whose relics were preserved in a bell-shaped shrine, and several kings of Ireland bore the associated name of Congal. In legend, Conall Cernach was a heroic warrior, who avenged the death of the Ulster champion, Cú Chulainn.

Conall Cernach

Connery

This comes from the Gaelic words for 'child of the hound' (hound, in this context, signifying a fierce warrior). It has become most familiar as a surname, although it is commonly used as a first name in the US. There are links with both Conroy and Conaire. The latter was particularly popular in ancient Ireland, where Conaire Mór was a renowned high king.

Connla

Meaning 'great chief', Connla (pronounced *KON-la*) figures prominently in early Irish lore. He was the son of Cú Chulainn, tragically slain by his father in a duel. Another Connla gave his name to a fabuous well, which bestowed great wisdom upon all who drank from its waters. Magical salmon swam in it, before transporting its knowledge to all the rivers of Ireland.

Connla,
son of Cú Chulainn

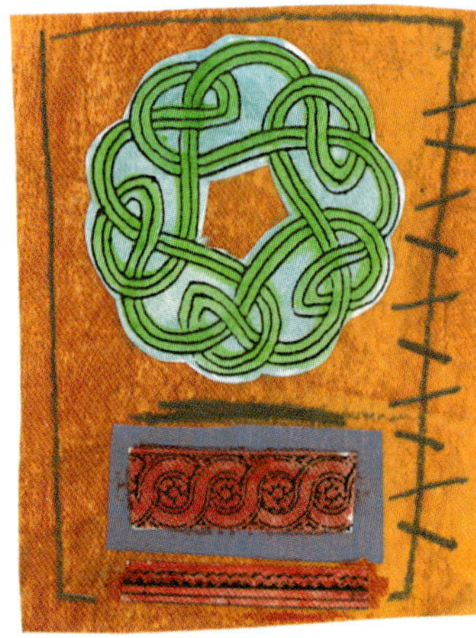

Connor, Conor

A contraction of Conchobar, a mythical king of ancient Ulster. He had the power of prophecy and carried an enchanted shield, which screamed aloud when anyone threatened him. Conchobar ruled over the Red Branch Knights, but his greatest warrior was his foster-son, Cú Chulainn. Both men featured in the early Irish epic, The Cattle Raid of Cooley, which described a war between Ulster and Connaught. Conchobar is sometimes regarded as a prototype for King Arthur.

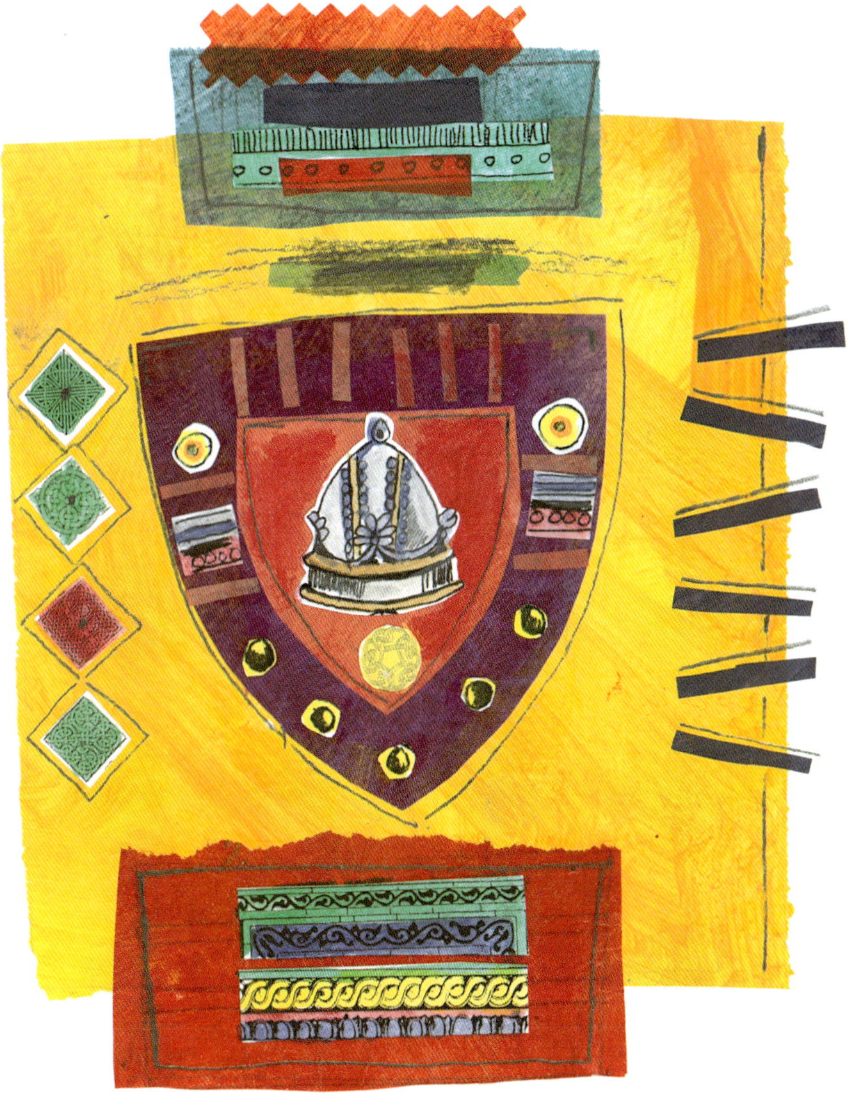

Conchobar,
mythical king of ancient Ulster

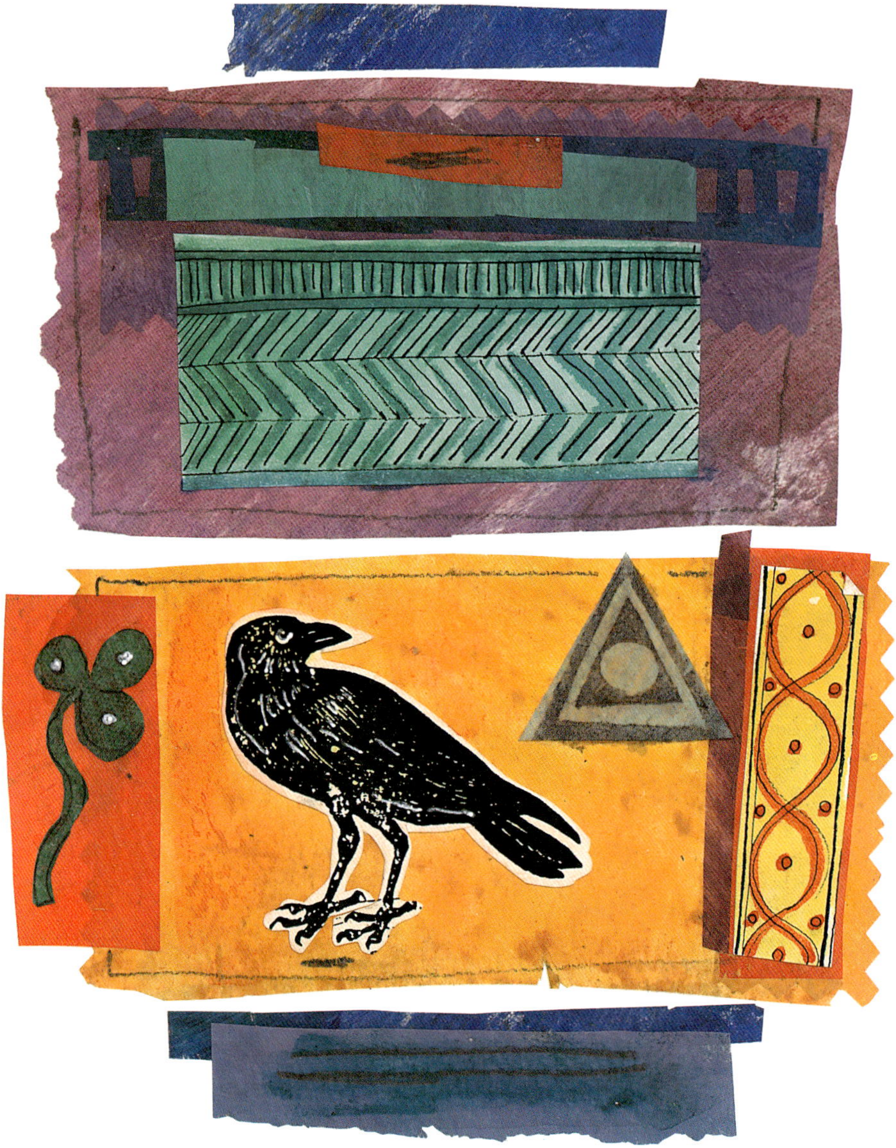

Cormac mac Airt, 3rd century AD

Cormac

A famous name in Irish legend, largely due to Cormac mac Airt, one of the first high kings. He was said to have ruled at Tara in the 3rd century AD but it is impossible to know if he was a genuine, historical figure. In the early sagas, he was portrayed as a wise man, an Irish King Arthur, presiding over Tara at the very time when the Fianna were performing some of their most spectacular exploits. Cormac was also involved in his own adventures. In one of these, he travelled to the Otherworld and won a magical bough from the sea-god, Manannán mac Lir. In later life, he was forced to abdicate after losing an eye – a tragic wound since, by law, no man could rule as high king if he suffered from a physical blemish.

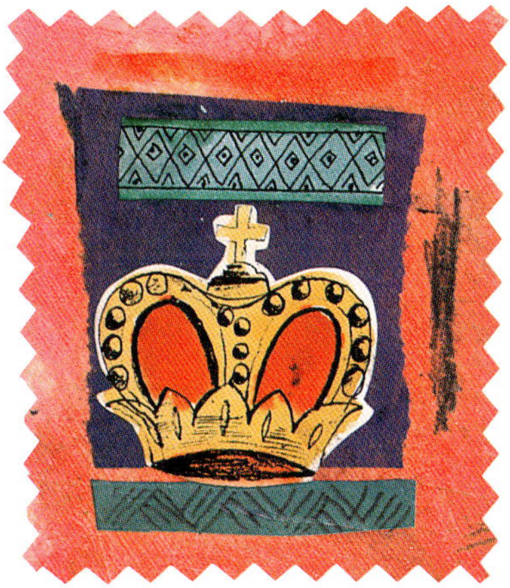

Cormac, Irish King Arthur

Curran

Deriving from the Gaelic word for 'hero' or 'champion', Curran is best known as a surname. In the Middle Ages, the O'Currans were a notable ecclesiastical family, headed by Simon O'Curran (d.1302), who became Bishop of Kilfenora. In recent years, Curran has found increasing favor as a first name.

D

Darragh

Darragh (pronounced *DAR-a*) comes from a Gaelic word meaning 'like an oak'. It is also an anglicized form of Dáire ('fertile'), a name which featured prominently in ancient legend. In the epic tale of *The Cattle Raid of Cooley*, Dáire mac Fiachna owned the magical bull which sparked off a war between Ulster and Connaught.

Dáire mac Fiachna, owner of the magical bull

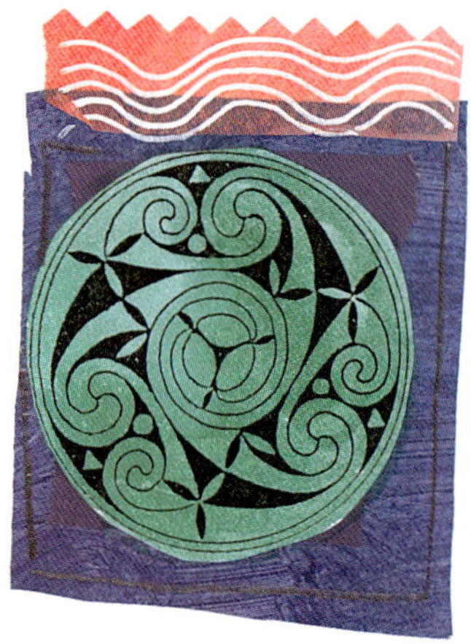

Darren

An Irish name meaning 'small and mighty'. Initially used as a surname, it gained wider currency in the US as a first name. There, it was promoted by the actor Darren McGavin (1922–) and by a character in the 1960s' television series *Bewitched*. Subsequently, it has become much more popular in Ireland and the UK, while its use in the US has declined.

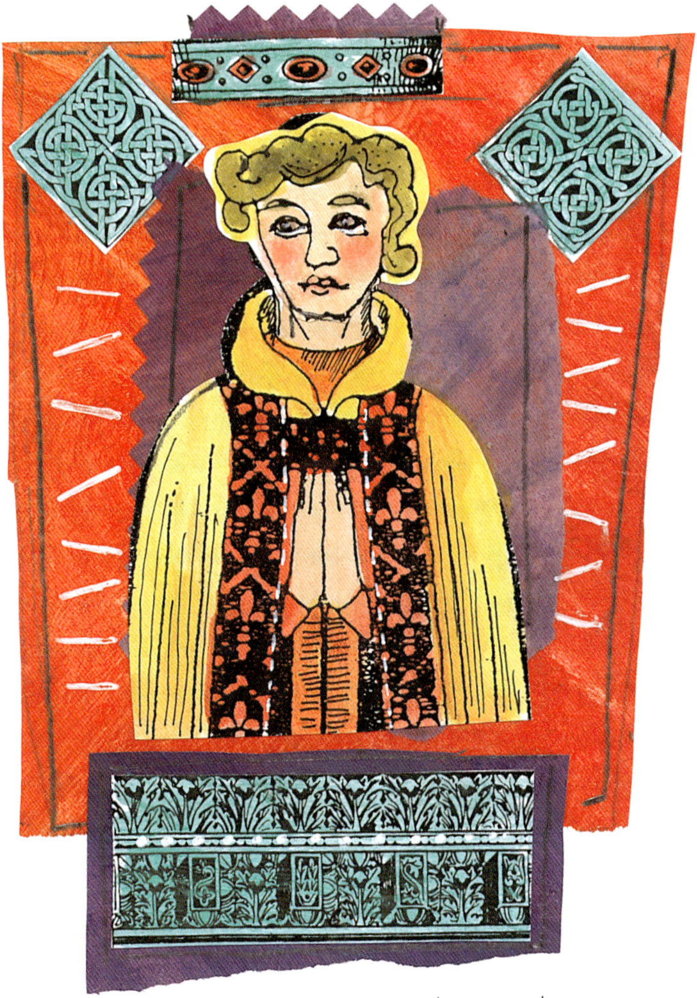

St. Declan, 5th century AD

DECLAN

DECLAN ('FULL OF GOODNESS') was one of the first Irish saints. He is said to have lived in the early 5th century, and to have begun his missionary work before the arrival of St. Patrick. He is usually cited as the founder of an important monastery at Ardmore, Co. Waterford, where several ancient monuments still bear his name.

Delany

Initially more popular as a surname, this is now finding increasing favor as a first name. It comes from the Irish word for 'challenger' or 'son of the champion'. There are also links with Delano, a French name meaning 'of the night', though this refers to the time of birth and has no sinister overtones.

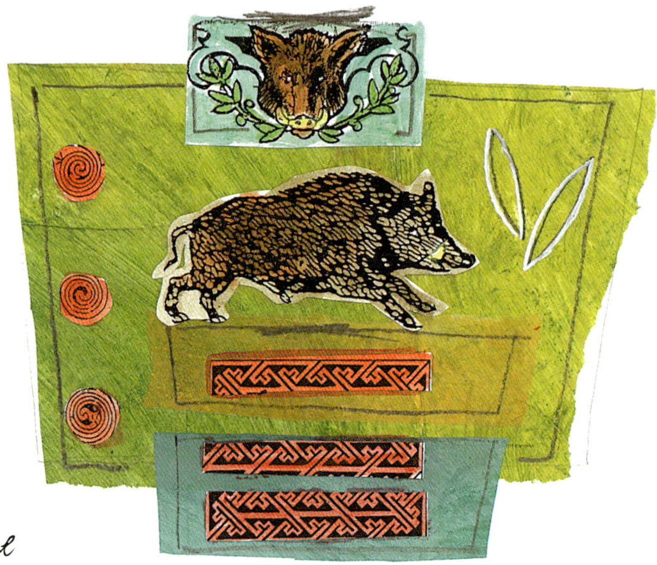

Diarmait Ua Duibhne

Dermot, Diarmait

A very popular name in ancient Ireland, borne by a host of early kings and legendary heroes. The most famous example of the latter was Diarmait Ua Duibhne, who had a love spot which made him irresistible to women. He eloped with Gráinne, the king's bride, and was pursued throughout Ireland for 16 years. He died on the slopes of Ben Bulben, after being gored by a magical boar.

Gerald, 3rd Earl of Desmond
(1338–98)

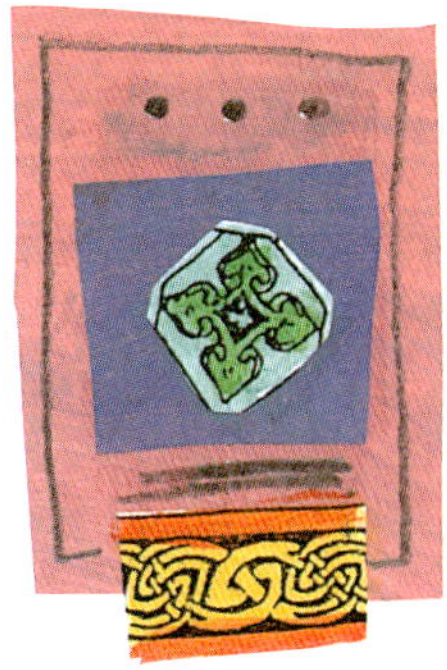

Desmond

This specified a man from southern Munster (*Deas Mumhan*) and it became the name of a territorial division there, in the days before the county system was devised. It is closely associated with the Fitzgerald family, who fought against English rule, most notably Gerald, 3rd Earl of Desmond (1338–98).

Dillon

This is thought to derive from *dealán* ('a streak of light'), although it may also have come from an Irish word for 'faithful'. It is often associated with the Welsh name, Dylan, which originally described a minor sea-god. Both in its Irish and Welsh forms, the name was quite uncommon until the poet, Dylan Thomas (1914–53) brought it international renown.

Donal

This was a very popular name in ancient Ireland, where its most common form was Domhnall. It means 'mighty ruler', which is highly appropriate, since it was the name of several Irish kings. Domnall Brecc (d.642) ruled Dalriada, an Irish enclave in Scotland, while his contemporary, Domnall, son of Aed, was the Irish high king and victor at the Battle of Moira (637).

DONAHUE, DONOGHUE

THIS STEMS FROM Donnchadh ('brown-haired warrior'), which was a popular name in medieval Ireland. Brian Boru (d.1014), the most famous of the high kings, had a son with this name. Donoghue became more familiar as a surname ('son of Donnchadh'), but it is now used increasingly as a first name in the US.

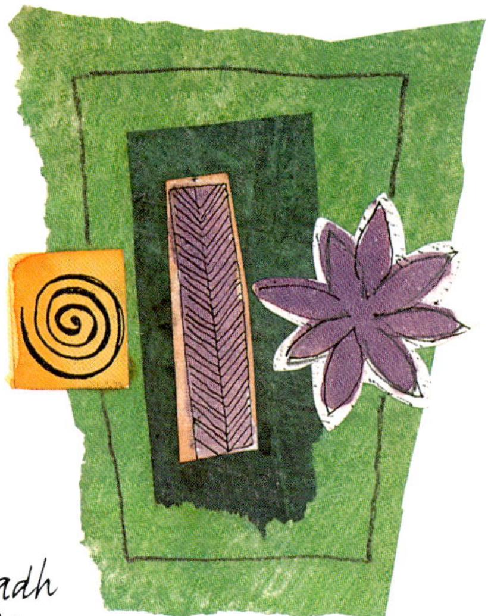

Donahue, from Donnchadh ('brown-haired warrior')

DONOVAN

LIKE DONOGHUE, Donovan stems from the ancient name of Donnchadh, which means 'brown-haired warrior'. It has been used both as a first name and as a surname, although the latter is probably more common. It gained a new lease of life as a first name in the 1960s, following the success of the Scottish folksinger Donovan Leitch (1946–).

E

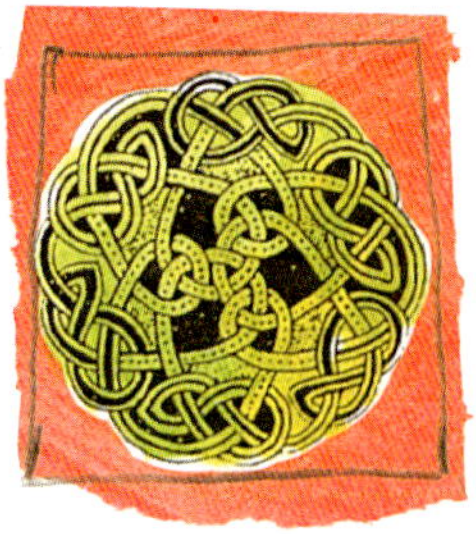

Eamon

Eamon (pronounced *EY-MON*) is an Irish form of Edmund, which was introduced into Ireland by the Anglo-Normans. It stems from *ead* ('riches') and *mund* ('guardian'). In the 20th century, the name is most closely associated with Eamon de Valera (1882–1973), who founded the Fianna Fáil party and became President of Ireland, and with the broadcaster Eamon Andrews (1922–87).

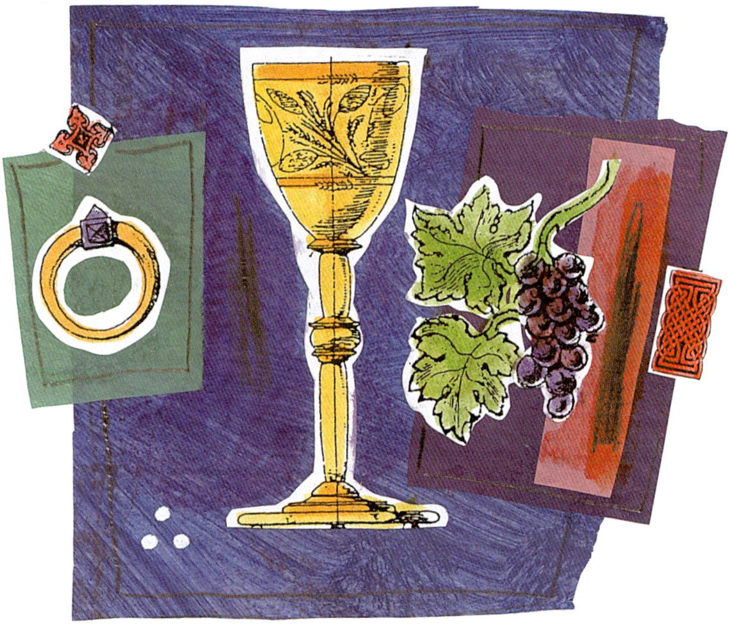

Eamon de Valera (1882–1973)

Eoghan

THE COLORFUL MEANING of this name (pronounced *OWEN*) is 'born of the yew tree'. It was extremely popular in early Irish history, both among warriors and saints. In the south, the Eóganachta ('people of Eógan) were a powerful ruling dynasty in Munster, while in the north the descendants of Eógan mac Néill gave their name to Tyrone (Tír Eógain or 'Land of Eógan).

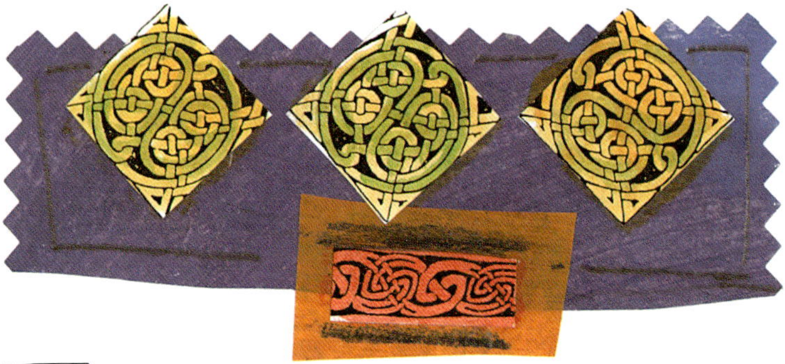

F

Faolan

PRONOUNCED *FWEEL-AWN*, this is thought to derive either from *fáel* ('a wolf') or *faolán* ('a seagull'). Fáelán was the warrior-son of Fionn mac Cumhaill, the leader of the Fianna. On a more peaceful note, St. Fillan (fl. early 8th century) was an Ulsterman, who became a missionary in Scotland. Robert the Bruce took his arm-relic to the Battle of Bannockburn (1314) and firmly believed that the saint was responsible for his victory.

Feabhal

This is a very ancient name (pronounced *FE-owl*) which features extensively in early Irish mythology, although mostly in association with minor characters. One of these was the father of Bran, the adventurer who travelled to the Otherworld. Another was a knight of the Fianna, the heroic war-band who were led by Fionn mac Cumhaill.

Ferdy

This is linked with the name Ferdiad ('man of smoke'), which figures prominently in early legend. In *The Cattle Raid of Cooley*, Ferdiad was the friend and foster-brother of Cú Chulainn. The pair trained together as warriors under Scáthach, the Amazonian queen of Skye, but they were later compelled to fight a bitter duel, in which Ferdiad was killed.

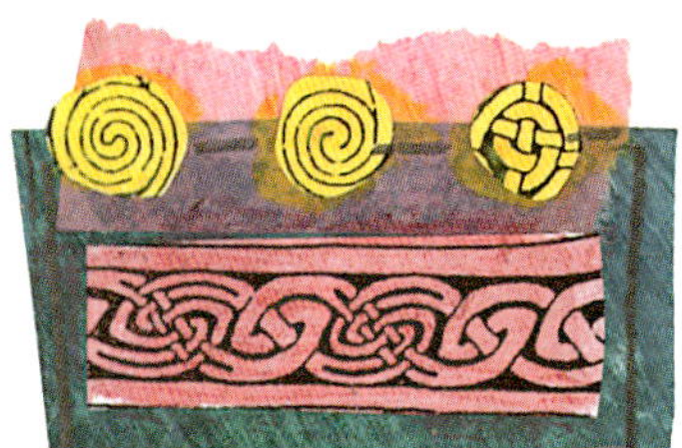

Fergal

Deriving from a word for 'valorous', Fergal was a popular name in early myth and history. The best-known example was Fergal mac Máeldúin, who ruled at Tara in the 8th century. He was the scourge of the Leinstermen, inflicting a number of defeats upon them, before they slew him at the Hill of Allen and placed his severed head upon a pike.

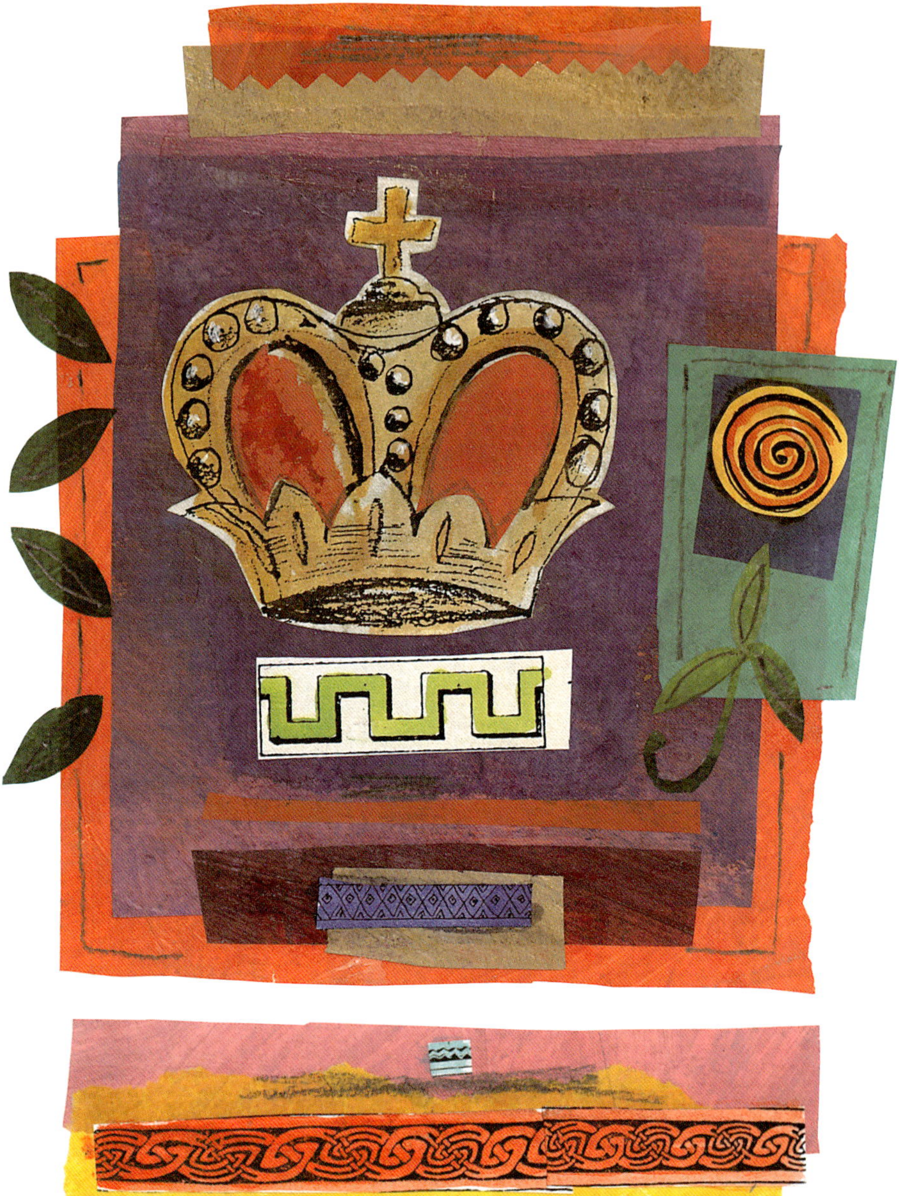

Fergus mac Roth

Fergus

One of the most popular Irish names, this probably derives from a word for 'virility'. There were many legendary kings and heroes with this name, the most famous being Fergus mac Roth. In *The Cattle Raid of Cooley*, he was duped out of the throne of Ulster by Nessa, his scheming lover. She agreed to marry Fergus, but only if he allowed her son Conchobar to rule in his place for twelve months. He consented, only to find himself banished from Ulster. He formed an alliance with Queen Maeve of Connaught and took up arms against his native land. However, he remained loyal to his foster-son, Cú Chulainn, and assisted him in the final, crucial battle.

Finbar

This is one of several Irish names which means 'fair-haired'. St. Finbar (c.560–c.610), the son of a blacksmith and a slave-girl, lived as a hermit, before founding a monastery at Cork. Finnbheara was the king of the Connaught fairies and the focus of many folk-tales. Described by some as the Irish Santa Claus, he was also feared as the lord of the dead.

Fingal

In ancient folklore, Fingal (literally the 'fair foreigner') was a powerful giant who built a bridge linking Ireland with the Hebrides, so that he could visit his fairy lover. The Irish end of this bridge was the Giant's Causeway, and it spanned the sea to Fingal's Cave on the island of Staffa. There was also a historical figure called Fingal, who became king of the Isle of Man (1070–7).

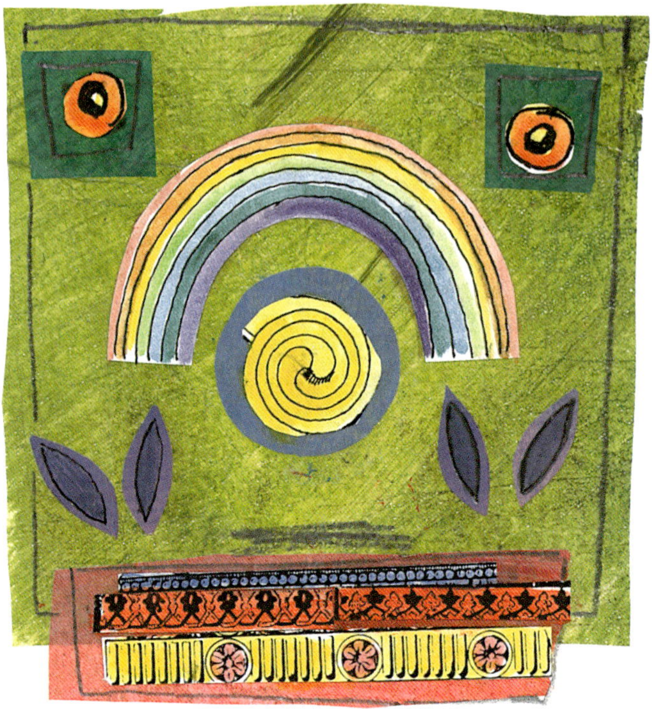

Finnian of Clonard
(d.549)

FINNIAN

MEANING 'FAIR-HAIRED', this name is most closely associated with two famous saints. Finnian moccu Telduib (d.549) is generally known as Finnian of Clonard, after the monastery in Co. Meath which he founded. He became renowned as a teacher, earning the nickname of the 'tutor of the saints of Ireland', and he is also cited as the author of the oldest surviving Irish penitential (a book listing the appropriate penance for each sin). Finnian of Moville (died c.579) is said to have taught St. Columba. According to legend, he was wooed by a Pictish princess. In recent times, the name has gained publicity from the film *Finian's Rainbow* (1968), which starred Fred Astaire.

Fintan

Official records list no fewer than 74 saints bearing the name of Fintan. These include Fintan of Clonenagh (d.603), who lived on a diet of barley-bread and water, and the much-travelled Fintan of Rheinau (d.879), who was enslaved by the Vikings, taken to the Orkneys and later became a hermit on the Rhine. In legend, Fintan was also the name of the only Irishman to survive the Biblical flood.

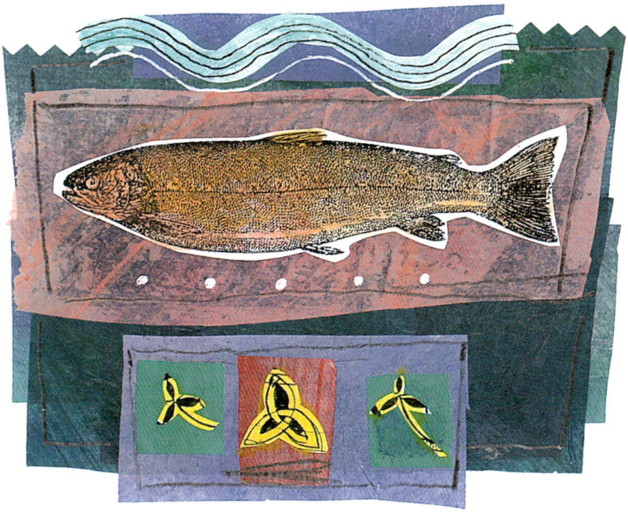

Fionn mac Cumhaill, leader of the Fianna

Fionn, Finn

Pronounced *FE-UN* this one of the greatest names in mythology. Fionn mac Cumhaill was the leader of the Fianna, Ireland's famous war-band. He acquired divine wisdom by eating the Salmon of Knowledge. This Otherworldly creature would impart its gifts if eaten in its entirety by a single person. Finnegas the Druid caught it, but his pupil, Fionn, inadvertently tasted a morsel and was allowed to claim it.

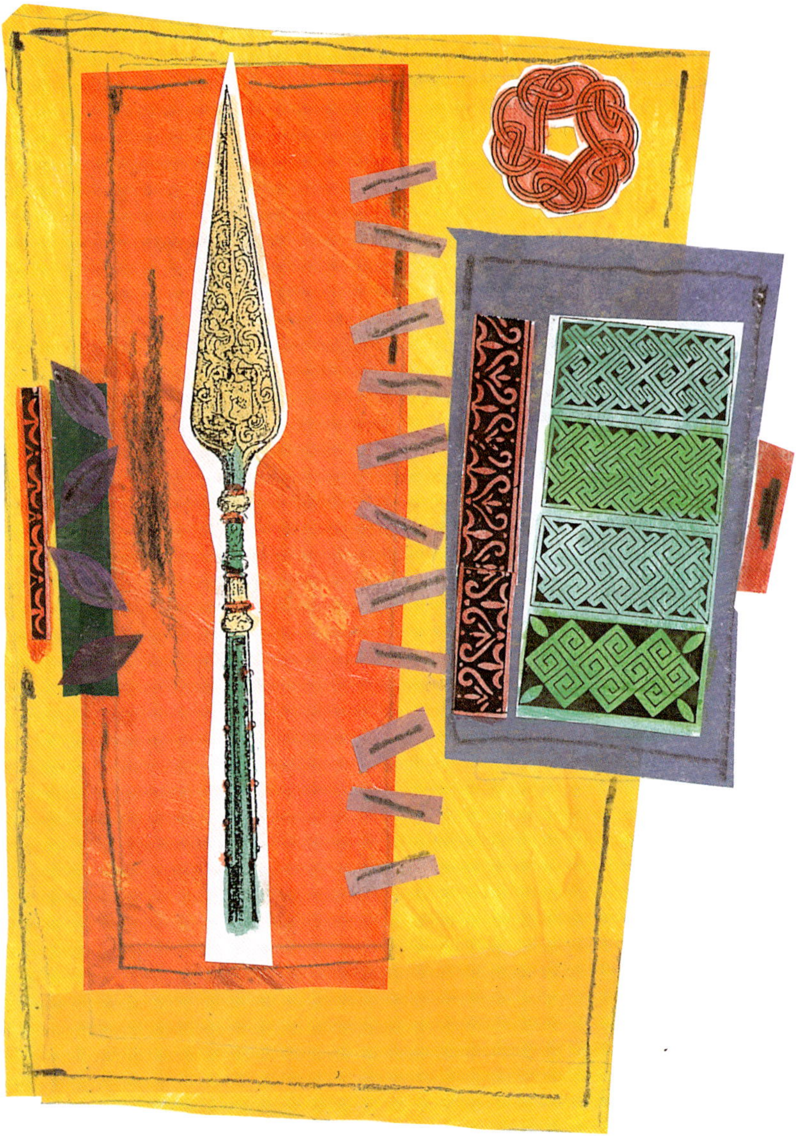

Gerald, 3rd Earl of Desmond
(1338–98)

Flann

Meaning 'bright red', this was a popular name for both boys and girls in ancient Ireland. Historically, its main association is with the poet, Flann mac Lonáin (fl. 9th/10th century). His satires were so vicious that they earned him the nickname of the 'Devil's Son', but his eloquence was equally legendary. At his funeral, it is said, he rose up to declaim a eulogy both for himself and for five others, who were buried on the same day.

Flann mac Lonáin (fl. 9th/10th century AD)

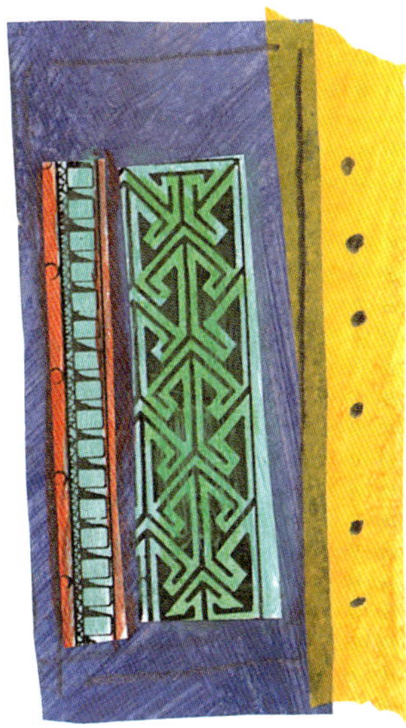

G

Gerald, Garrett

This ancient name has Teutonic origins and means 'spear-might'. It was introduced into Ireland by the Anglo-Normans and was closely associated with the Fitzgerald family, most notably Gerald, 3rd Earl of Desmond (1338–98). He was believed to have magical powers, which enabled him to climb into a bottle or shape-shift into a bird. Some say that he is sleeping at the bottom of Lough Gur, waiting to return to the land of the living.

K

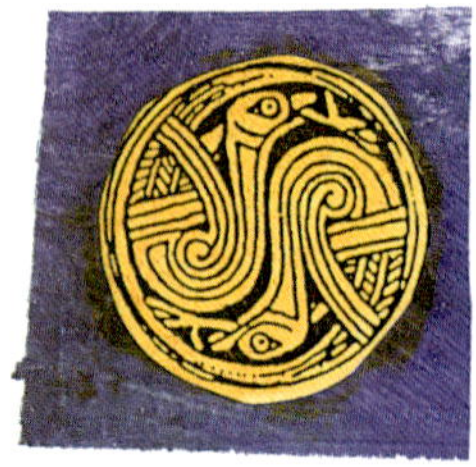

Kermit, Kermode

Of Irish or Manx origin, this unusual name evolved from a shortening of the surname, MacDermot. One of the sons of the US President, Theodore Roosevelt (1858–1919), was called Kermit, but the name has declined in popularity in recent years, partly because of its strong associations with Kermit the Frog in *The Muppet Show*.

Kevin

This stems from the Irish word *caoimhín*, meaning 'comely child'. St. Kevin (d.618) was one of Ireland's most famous saints. Born into a noble Leinster family, he lived as a hermit before founding the monastery of Glendalough (Co. Wicklow). With its lofty round tower, this is one of the nation's most beautiful landmarks. Kevin was a great animal-lover. While living as an anchorite, he was fed by an otter, which used to bring him salmon each day. On one occasion, a blackbird laid an egg in his hand while his arms were outstretched in prayer. With great patience, he held it there until the egg hatched out.

St. Kevin, lived as an anchorite

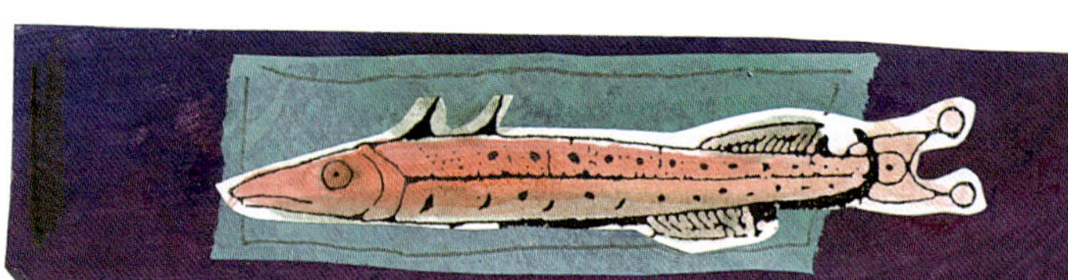

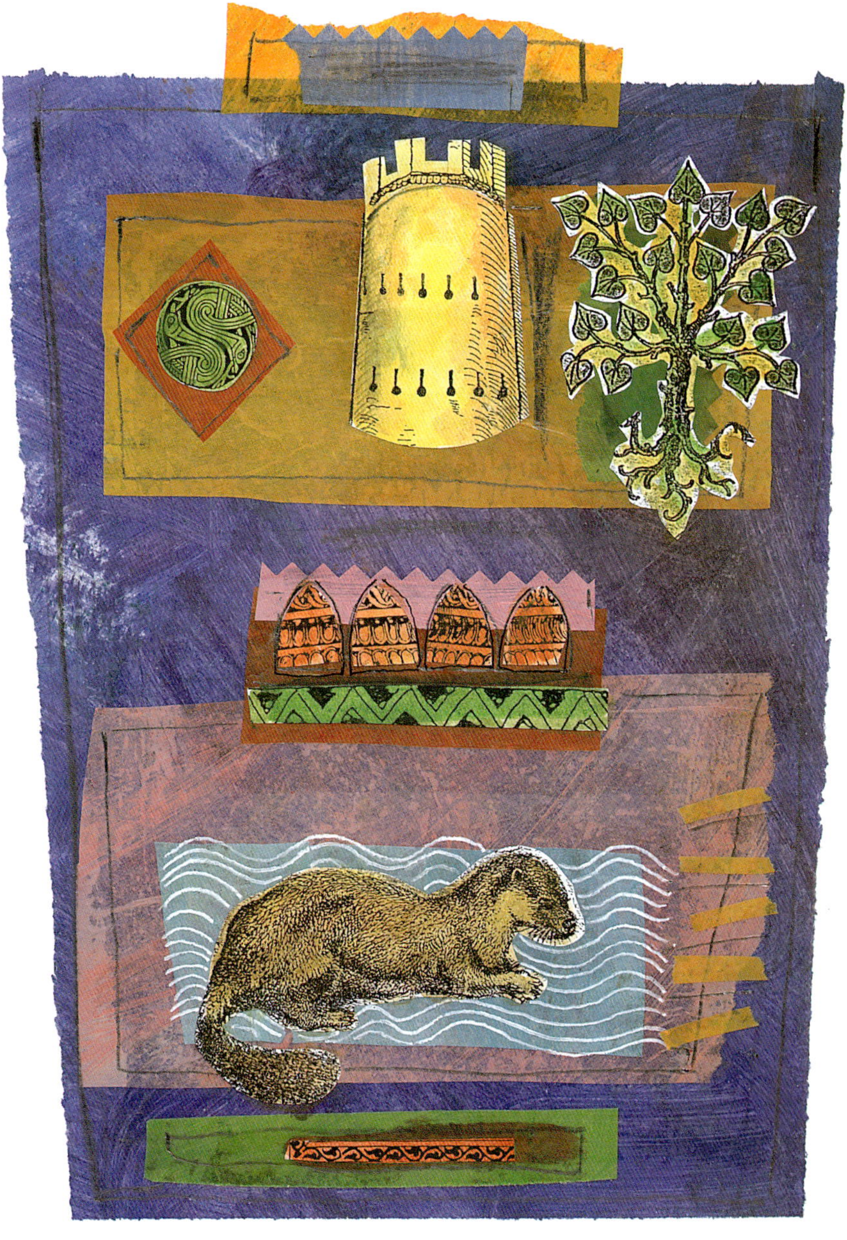

St. Kevin (d.618),
one of Ireland's most famous saints

Kieran, Ciarán

Now becoming increasingly popular, this name comes from *ciar* ('black'). It is chiefly associated with St. Ciarán (c.512–c.545), who founded the monastery of Clonmacnois, which boasts a glorious collection of Celtic crosses. According to legend, *The Cattle Raid of Cooley* was dictated to the saint and one of the oldest surviving manuscripts of the text, The Book of the Dun Cow (c.1100), was written on the hide of his cow. St. Ciarán of Saighir (5th/6th century) founded a monastery, the resting place of the kings of Ossory.

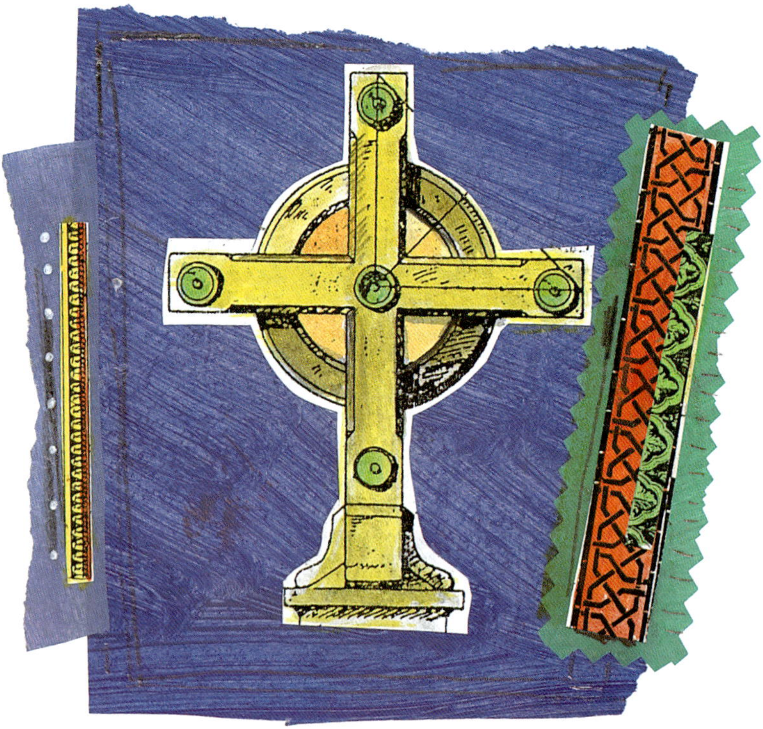

St. Ciarán (c.512–c.545),
founder of the monastery of Clonmacnois

Killian

The name is thought to derive from *cill* ('a monk's cell') and, not surprisingly perhaps, it is linked with several saints. The best-known was a 7th-century Irishman, who carried out missionary work in the Rhine area. He became Bishop of Würzburg after converting the local chieftain from paganism, but met a violent death when intervening in a marriage dispute. He was included in Irish martyrologies from the 9th century, but is principally known as the patron saint of Würzburg. The city celebrates a *Kilianfest* each year, when mystery plays are performed.

Killian,
Bishop of Würzburg

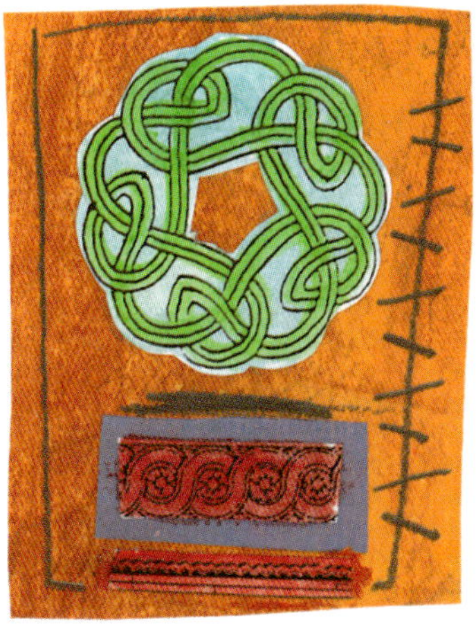

L

Laoghaire

The origin of this name, pronounced *LAY-ora*, is uncertain, although it may mean 'calf-herd'. Several high kings were called Laoghaire, the most famous of these being the son of Niall of the Nine Hostages. His reign coincided with the arrival of St. Patrick in Ireland, and he became one of the saint's first converts. The name is preserved in the resort of Dún Laoghaire, Co. Dublin.

LIAM

A SHORTENED FORM of William ('will' and 'helmet'), this was introduced to Ireland by the Anglo-Normans. For centuries it was used only as a pet name, gaining widest currency as *Liam na Lasoige* ('Will-o'-the-wisp'). Now popular in its own right, it has been made fashionable by figures such as Liam Neeson (actor), Liam Gallagher (rock musician) and Liam Cosgrave (politician).

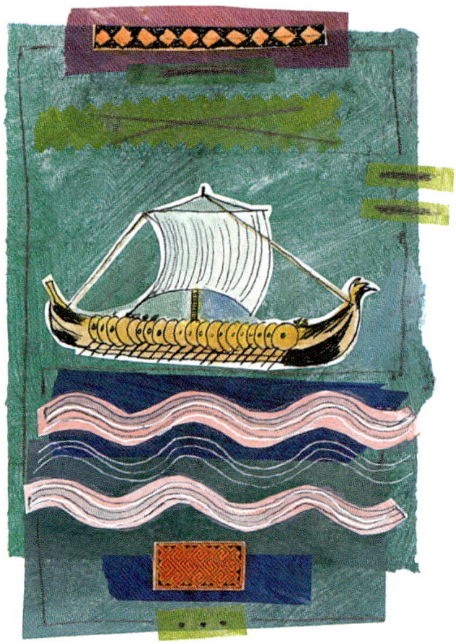

MacLochlainne, 'Son of the Norseman'

LOCHLAN, LOCHLANN

THIS NAME, PRONOUNCED *LOK-LUN*, used to strike fear into Irish hearts, for Lochlann (literally 'Lakeland') was the home of the Viking raiders, who caused devastation during the 9th and 10th centuries. Once they began to settle in Ireland and intermarry, however, MacLochlainne ('Son of the Norseman') became a popular name.

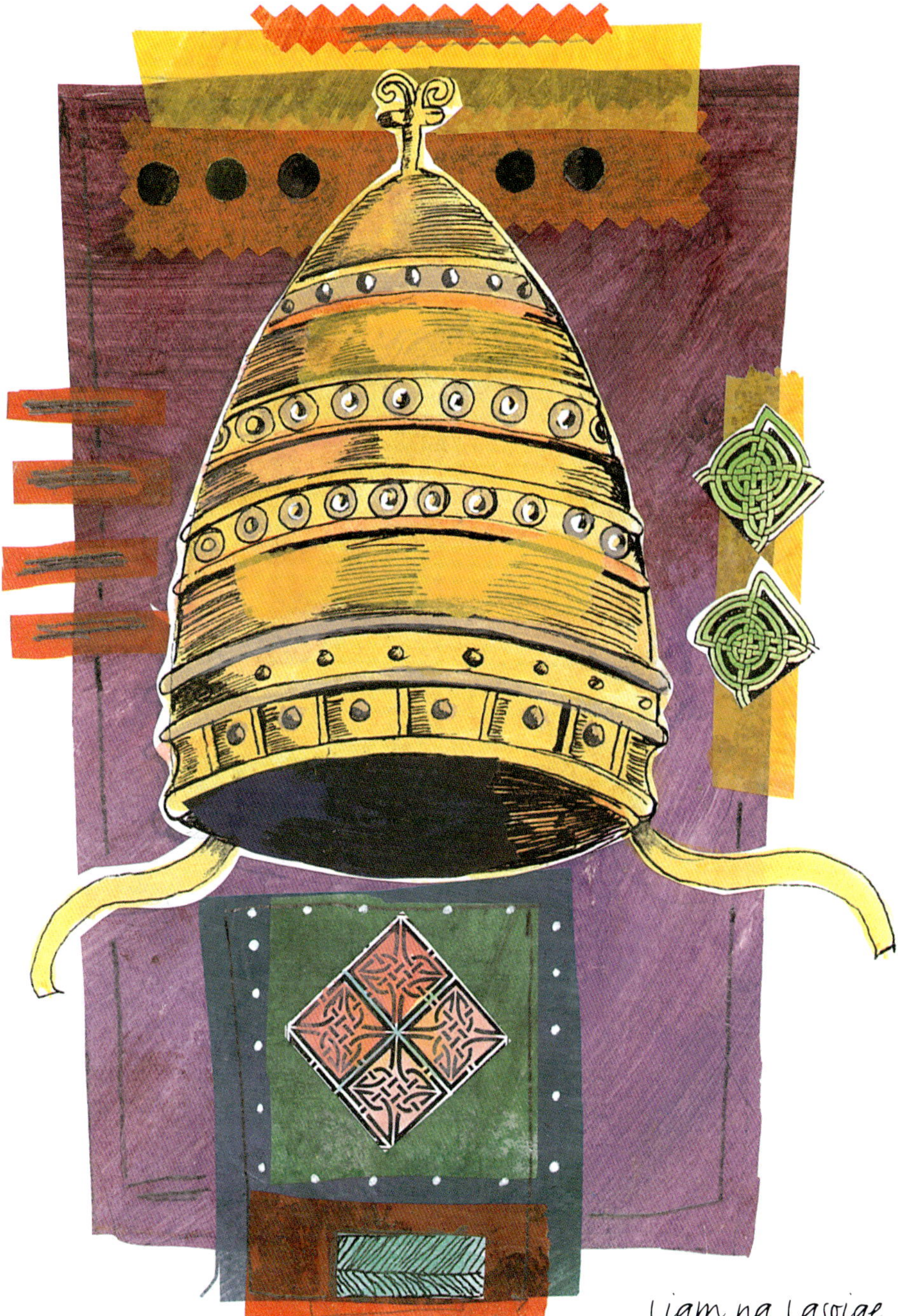

Liam na Lasoige

Lorcan

This ancient name, pronounced *LOR-KAN,* is a diminutive of *lorc* ('fierce') and was traditionally used for the sons of warriors. Its chief association is with a churchman – Lorcán Ua Tuathail, who is anglicized as Laurence O'Toole (1128–80). He became Archbishop of Dublin in 1162 and frequently mediated between the Irish and the English. He was canonized in 1225.

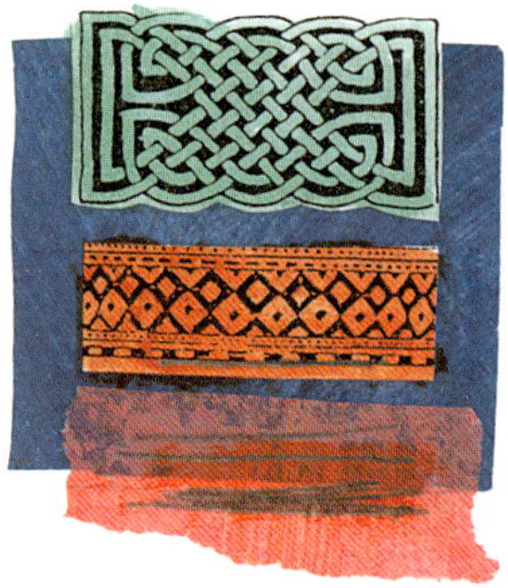

M

Malachy

This name has a dual origin. The influential Archbishop of Armagh, St. Malachy (1094–1148) adopted it from the Old Testament prophet, Malachi (literally 'my angel'). In addition, it is linked with an Irish king, Maoilseachlainn, which means 'follower of St. Seachlainn'. The latter, who is better known by the Latinized form 'Secundinus', was one of the first missionaries in Ireland.

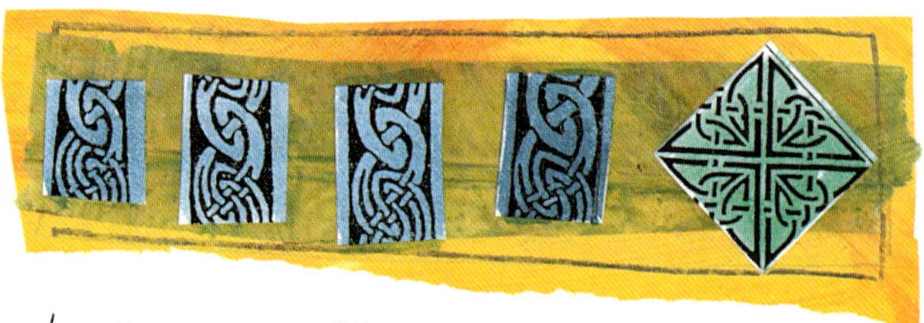

St. Malachy (1094–1148)

Michael

Michael is a biblical name, deriving ultimately from the Hebrew Micah ('who is like God'). In this context, its closest links are with the archangel and weigher of souls at the Last Judgment. The cult of St. Michael was very strong in Ireland, as the monastic settlement of Skellig Michael (Co. Kerry) confirms. More recently, the name has been popularized by Mícheál mac Liammóir (1899–1978), the distinguished actor, playwright and director.

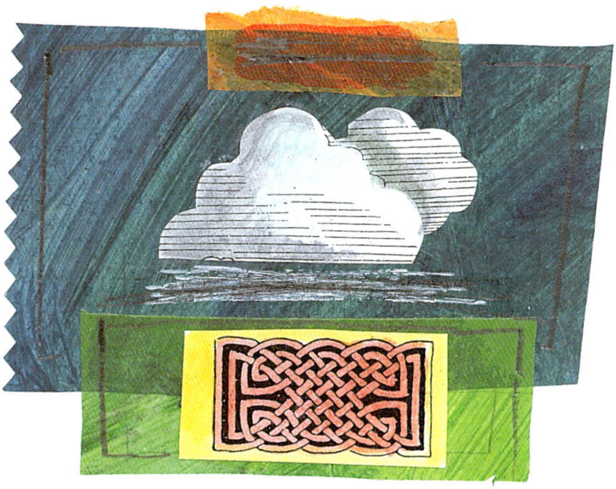

N

Niall

Niall of the Nine Hostages

Meaning either a 'cloud' or a 'champion', Niall (pronounced *KNEE-al*) is the Irish form of Neil. It is an ancient name, borne by several of the high kings at Tara. The most famous of these was Niall of the Nine Hostages, who is said to have ruled in the 4th century AD. His hostages came from the British, the French, the Scots, the Saxons and the five kingdoms of Ireland.

O

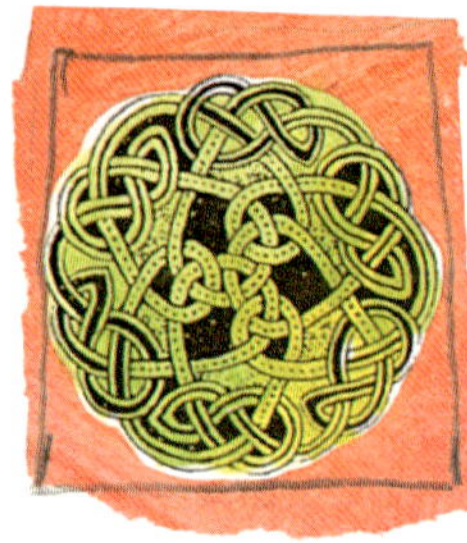

OISIN

PRONOUNCED *OSH-EEN*, this evocative name means 'little deer'. Its origin can be found in the legend of Oisin, who was the son of Fionn mac Cumhaill and one of the leading warriors in the Fianna. His mother, Sadb, was transformed into a doe by an evil druid, and the young Oisin was reared in the wild until he was seven years old.

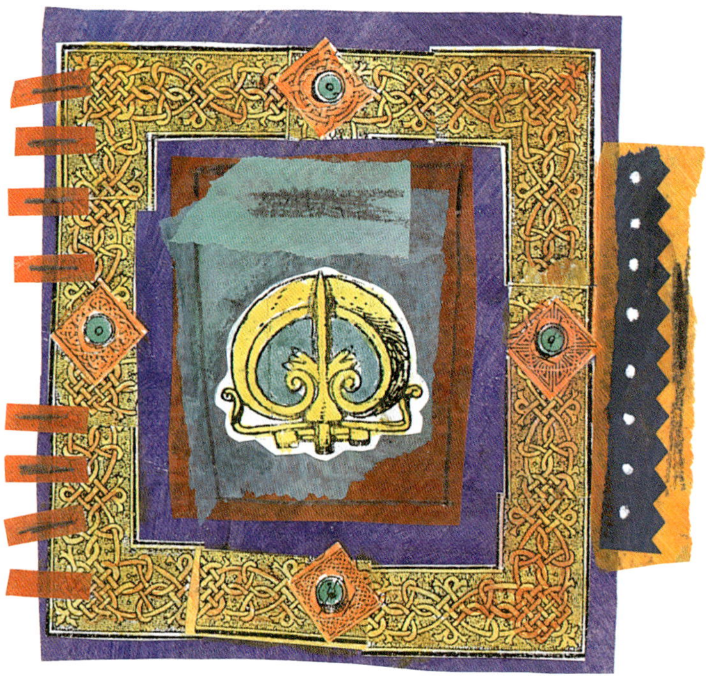

Oscar, son of Oisin
(a warrior)

Oscar

THE MOST CELEBRATED OSCAR in Irish legend was the son of Oisin and, as with his father, the name derives from *os* ('a deer'). Oscar went on to join the Fianna and become its most valorous warrior – the Irish equivalent of Sir Galahad. In one of the Christianized stories, he enabled his comrades to escape from hell. In modern times, the name was made famous by the author and wit, Oscar Wilde (1854–1900).

P

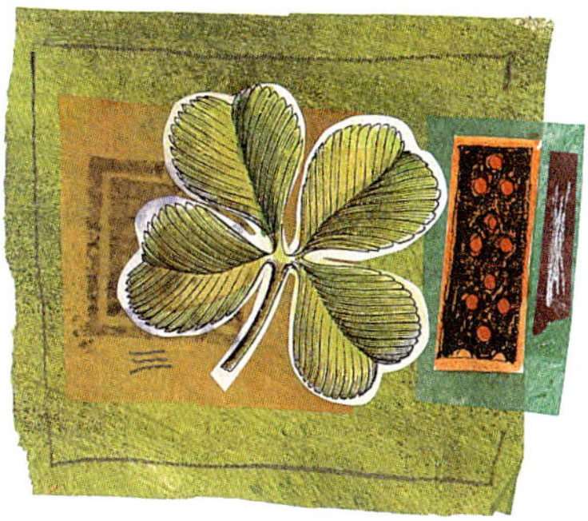

Partholon, Partlan

IN IRISH MYTHOLOGY, Partholon (pronounced *part-o-LAWN*) was the leader of an ancient race of invaders who settled in Ireland in Biblical times. Originally from the eastern Mediterranean, they were forced to flee from their native land after Partholon had murdered his father. Their wanderings lasted for seven years, before they finally arrived in Ireland. Despite Partholon's violent past, he and his people brought many benefits to their new home. They were said to have introduced agriculture, clearing the central plains of the forests and establishing the first farms, and also taught ale-brewing and cauldron-making. The name probably derives from the Aramaic word, Bartholomew.

Patrick,
patron saint of Ireland

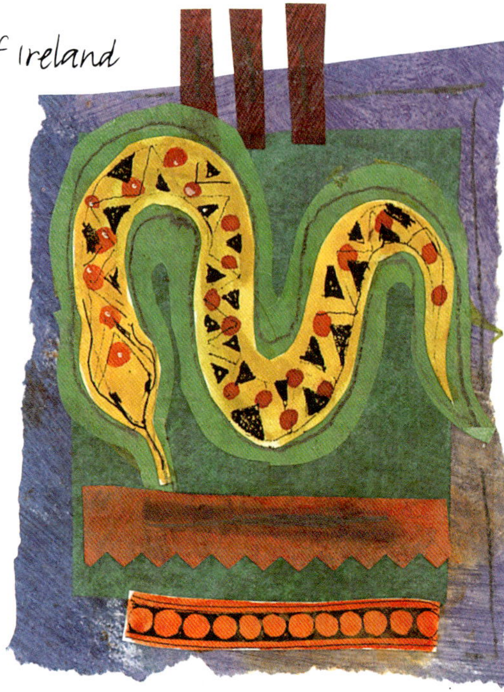

PATRICK, PADRAIG

PATRICK (c.390–461?), the patron saint of Ireland, was a Roman citizen living in the west of Britain during the twilight years of the Empire. In his youth, he was carried off to Ireland as a slave. He soon escaped to Gaul, where he studied for the priesthood. Then in c.432 he returned to Ireland as a missionary, beginning his ministry at Saul, Co. Down. Over the following years he managed to banish the snakes (i.e. heathenism) from much of the country and established his principal church at Armagh. According to legend, the key episode in the conversion process occurred at the mound of Tara in 432. There, on Easter Sunday, Patrick confronted the pagan high king and his druids, and lit the sacred flame of Christianity on the Hill of Slane.

R

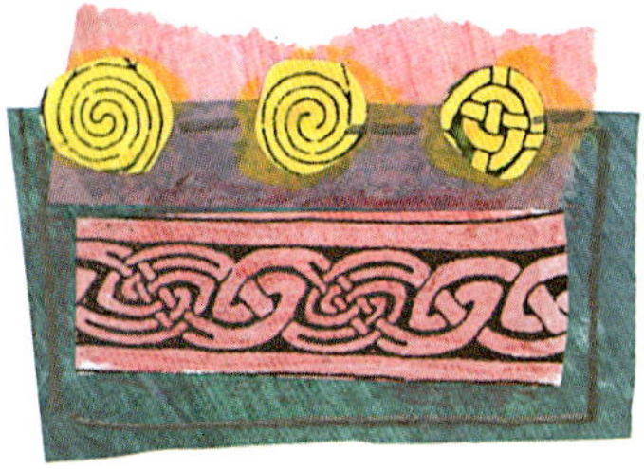

Ronan

THE NAME IS A DIMINUTIVE of *rón*, the Irish word for 'seal'. It is linked with a number of saints, several of whom have animal connections. One kept a pet wolf and was accused of being a werewolf himself, while another had a vision of riding upon a whale. Ronan the Silent was an Irish anchorite who led a mission to Brittany where his name is commemmorated in the town of Locronan. At Innerleithen in Scotland another St Ronan was said to have chased away the devil, a feat still celebrated in the annual 'St. Ronan's Games'. There are also possible links with St. Ruadán, who placed a curse on Tara and its druids.

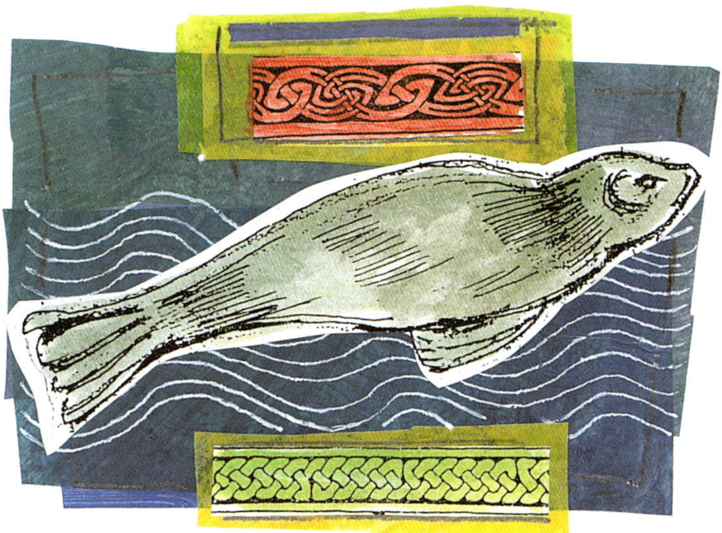

Ronan the Silent

Rory

From a Gaelic word meaning 'red king', this name is popular in both Ireland and Scotland. It was widely used in the Middle Ages, although its Irish associations are tinged with melancholy, since it was the name of the very last high king. Rory O'Connor was forced to abdicate in 1183 and retired to the Abbey of Cong. He died there 15 years later, a forgotten man.

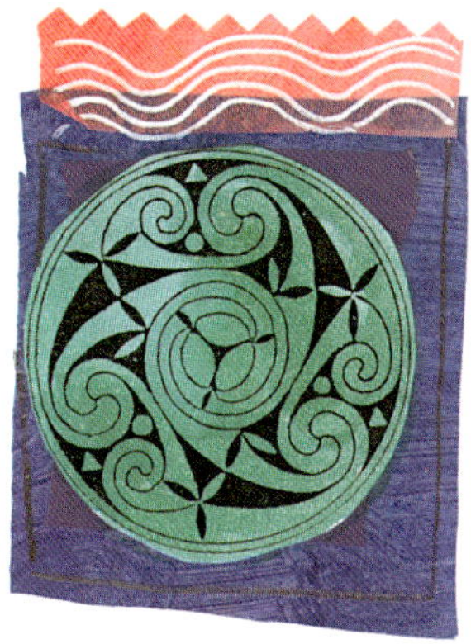

S

Seamus

In spite of its very strong Irish associations, the origins of this name are not Celtic. It is the Irish form of James, which means 'supplanter' and whose traditional emblem is a scallop shell. The name was extremely popular with the Anglo-Normans. James, Earl of Desmond, for example, was more commonly known as Séamus Iarla Deasmuman. There have been many famous Irishmen with this name. Seamus Murphy (1907–75) was a noted sculptor, who produced bronze busts of all the Presidents from Hyde to O'Dalaigh. Seamus Heaney (1939–), meanwhile, is an outstanding poet, renowned for such works as *Wintering Out* (1972) and *Station Island* (1984). The name is so evocative of Ireland that *shamus* has become American slang for a 'detective'.

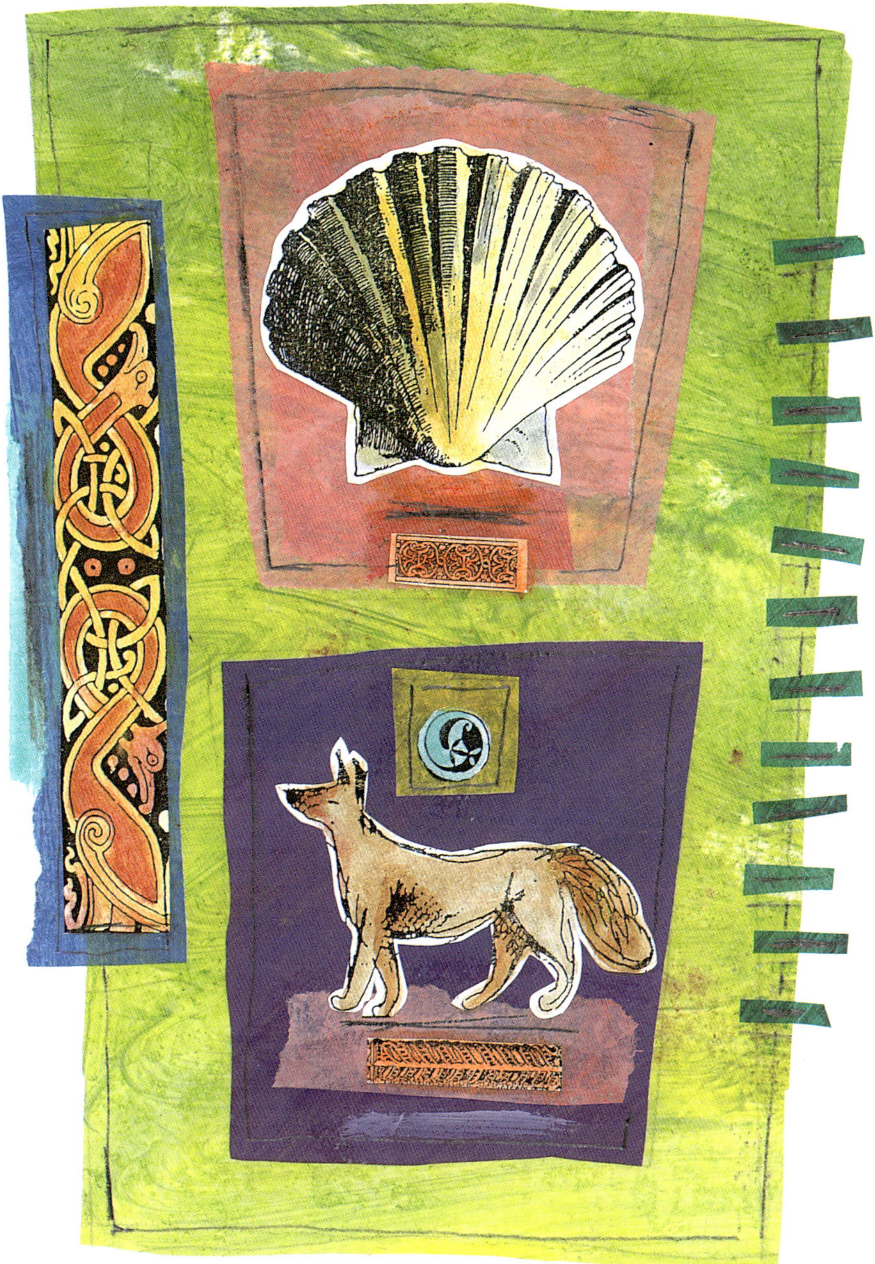

Séamus Iarla Deasmuman

SEAN

SEAN IS THE IRISH FORM OF JOHN, which means 'God's gracious gift'. It was introduced into Ireland by the Anglo-Normans, who spelt it *Jehan*. In the 16th century, Shane O'Neill won notable victories against the armies of Elizabeth I. More recently, the name has been popularized by the actors Sean Connery, Sean Bean and Sean Penn.

T

TURLOUGH

PRONOUNCED *TUR-LOK*, this is an anglicized form of *toirdhealbhach*, which means 'instigator'. It was a name shared by two of the last high kings, Turlough O'Brien (d.1086) and Turlough O'Connor (d.1156). Its most famous association, however, is with the harpist and composer, Turlough O'Carolan (1670–1732), who achieved great success, despite being blinded in his youth.

TYRONE

THIS COLORFUL NAME originated as a territorial division. Tír Eógain ('Land of Eógan') referred to the domain of a son of Niall of the Nine Hostages, who settled there in the 5th century AD. In modern times, the name was linked almost exclusively with two American actors, father and son, who were both named Tyrone Power (1869–1931 and 1913–58), but its use is now becoming much more widespread.

Girls' Names

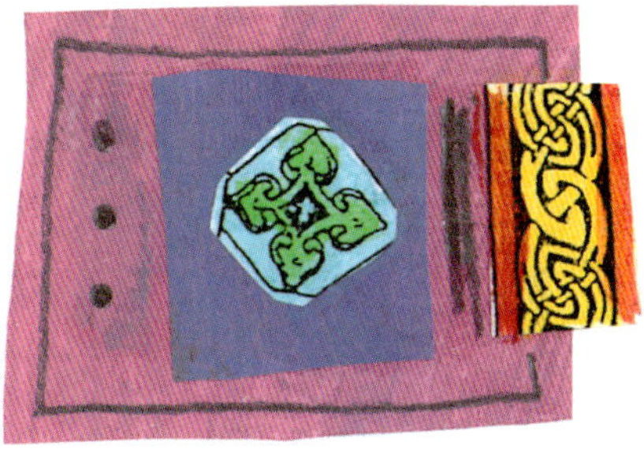

In the early days of Irish history, parents had to choose from a comparatively small selection of female names. Medieval sources list just 300 options for girls, while for boys there were around 3,000. As a result, a significant number of borrowings from other languages were made during the period of the invasions. Of the traditional Irish names, many can be traced back to ancient legend or folklore. Some, like Grania, Deirdre and Emer were the focus of great love stories, whilst others, such as Maeve and Aoife were renowned for their power and influence. Many were linked with goddesses, relating to nature and the land. Some rivers, for example, have become girls' names, because they were once believed to be the dwelling places of protective female spirits. In a similar vein, some names have come to be used as poetic symbols for the charm and beauty of Ireland itself.

A

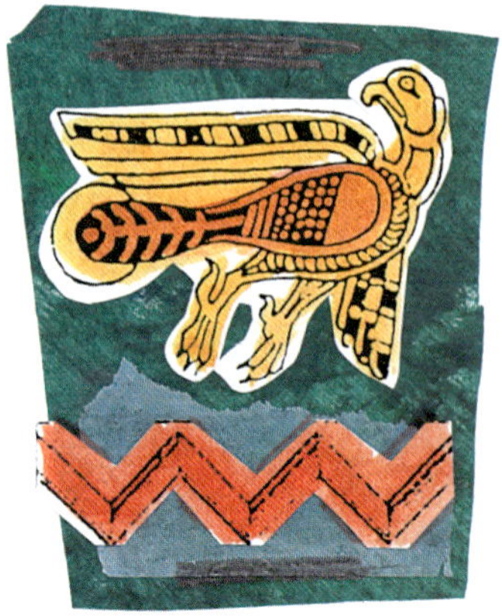

Alana, Alannah

THIS NAME IS POPULAR throughout the Celtic world from Brittany to Scotland, although its origin is uncertain. `It probably derives from the phrase *a leanbh*, a term of endearment which can roughly be translated as 'darling child'. Alternatively, it may have developed as a feminine form of Alan, itself from a Gaelic name which means 'handsome' or 'cheerful'. The name has several variants, most notably Alanis, which has been popularized in recent years by the Canadian singer, Alanis Morissette.

Alison

ALISON MAY DERIVE FROM a Gaelic word for 'small and truthful', but it is more likely that it developed as a diminutive form of Alice. This stemmed ultimately from a German term *adelheidis*, meaning 'of noble birth'. In France, this was shortened to Adaliz, before becoming Aliz. It was in this form that the Anglo-Normans introduced the name into Ireland and it can now be found in most Celtic areas. In recent times, it has been popularized by a number of writers, including Alison Uttley (1884–1976), Alison Lurie and Alison Fell.

Alma

THIS NAME HAS BEEN USED independently in several different cultures. In Hebrew, it means 'maiden'; in Spanish, it is a word for 'spirit' or 'soul'; and in Latin, it means 'kind' or 'nourishing'. The Celtic version of the name stems from Almha ('all good'), a minor Irish goddess, who was noted for her strength.

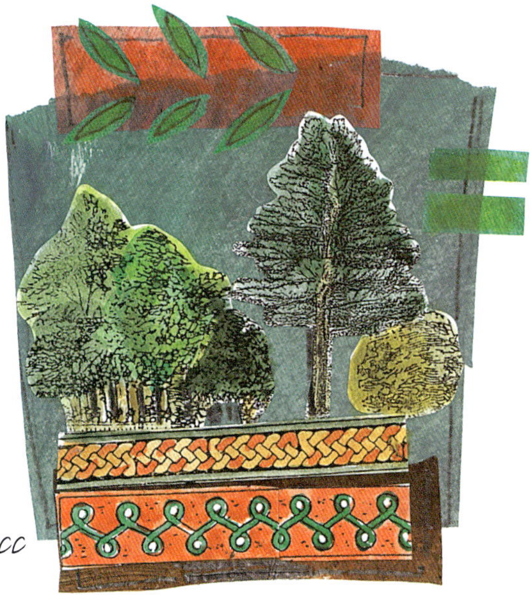

Ailbe Grúadbrecc

Alva

THIS IS AN anglicized form of Ailbe ('white'), a name that was popular for both boys and girls. Ailbe Grúadbrecc ('of the freckled cheeks') was a daughter of the high king, Cormac mac Airt, and was wooed by Fionn mac Cumhaill, who asked her to live with him in the forest. On the male side, St. Ailbe (early 6th century) was one of the first Irish missionaries, and was said to have been suckled by a she-wolf.

Aoibheann

Pronounced *EVE-een*, this comes from a Gaelic word meaning 'radiant beauty'. It was a common name among the royal families of early Irish history and there are also some ecclesiastical connections. The mother of St. Enda of Aran (died c.530) was called Aobhín. Today, the name is frequently anglicized as Eavan.

Aoife, warrior queen and lover of Cú Chulainn

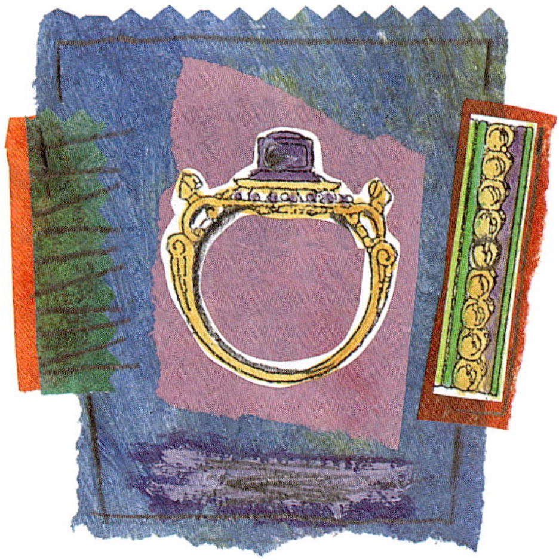

Aoife

Aoife (pronounced *EEF-a*) is a name with tragic associations in Irish legend. On the Island of Shadows, she was a warrior queen who lost her heart to Cú Chulainn and bore him a son named Connla. Years later, the latter was slain by his father, who realized his mistake when he recognized a thumb-ring, which he had given to the boy. More tragic still was the Aoife who fell in love with Ilbrec. She was transformed into a crane by a jealous rival and, after her death, her skin was used to make the Treasure Bag of the Fianna. The name has gained popularity since 1997, when the Siamese twins, Aoife and Niamh, were successfully separated.

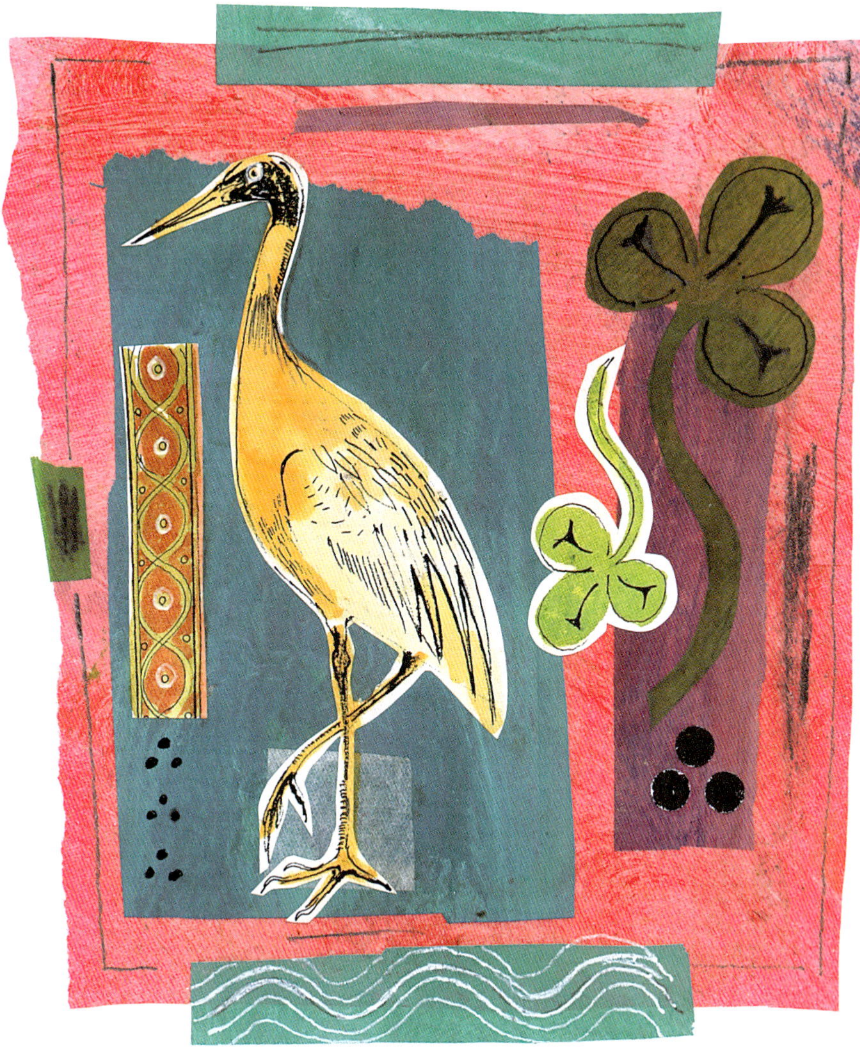

Aoife, who fell in
love with Ilbrec

Ashling, Aisling

This evocative name comes from a word meaning 'dream' or 'vision', and originally had patriotic overtones. It stems from a type of verse – usually known as 'Aisling poetry' – which was very popular in the 17th and 18th centuries. In this, the poet would be out walking in the countryside, when he came across a beautiful woman, who was the personification of Ireland.

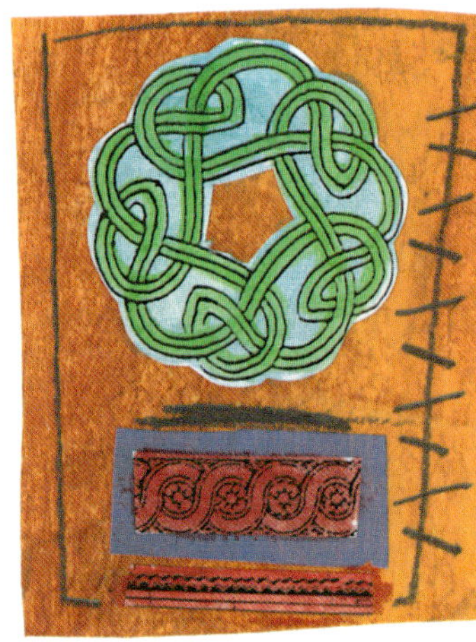

B

Bairbre

This is the Irish form of Barbara (pronounced *BARB-re*), a name which is derived from the Greek word for 'foreign woman'. The name became enormously popular in Ireland in the Middle Ages in response to the cult of St. Barbara. Legend relates how her father had her executed when she refused to give up her Christian faith, before he was, in turn, struck down by a bolt of lightning. As a result, St. Barbara became the patron saint of gunners, miners and firework-makers.

BERNADETTE

THIS IS THE FEMININE FORM of the French name, Bernard. It became a great favorite in Ireland, as a result of the popular cult of St. Bernadette (1844–79). At the age of 14 she experienced a series of visions of the Virgin Mary, which revealed the curative powers of a local spring at Lourdes. This has since become a major pilgrimage centre.

BRENDA

IT IS OFTEN ASSUMED that this name is simply a feminine form of Brendan, and that its success in Ireland was due to the immense popularity of St. Brendan the Navigator (c.486–c.575). In fact, it is more likely that the name was introduced by the Vikings, deriving from their word for 'bright sword'. The name has been made familiar in recent years by the actresses, Brenda Fricker and Brenda Blethyn.

BRENNA

THIS IS A FAIRLY modern name, principally used in the US. Its derivation is uncertain, although it is probably a feminine form of Bran. As such, its meaning would be 'beauty with hair as dark as a raven'. The other possibilities are that it stems from Briana (a female version of Brian), from the surname Branagh, or from the Welsh name Brynna ('a hill').

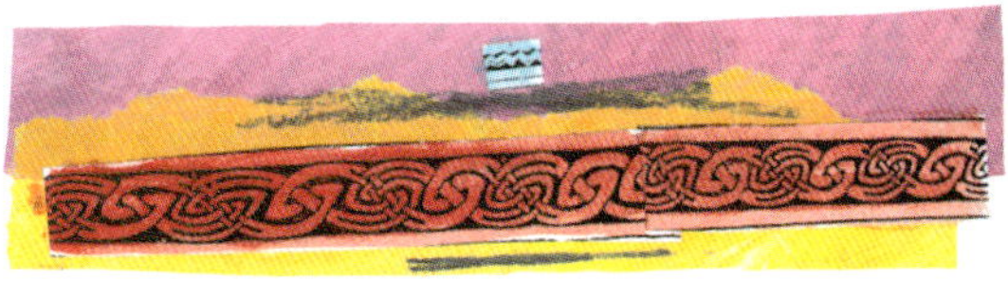

Brenna

Bridget, Brigid

Brigid was a Celtic fertility goddess, linked with healing and women in childbirth. Her cult was celebrated on 1st February, at the ancient pastoral festival of Imbolc, which marked the time when ewes came into milk. Many of the goddess's attributes were transferred to St. Brigid of Kildare (c.450–c.523), during the early Christian period. According to tradition, she was raised in a druid's household and was fed with the milk of Otherworld cows. In reality, she founded the monastery of Kildare and her reputation in Ireland was second only to that of St. Patrick. Indeed, there is a legend that the two saints were buried in the same tomb in Downpatrick (Co. Down).

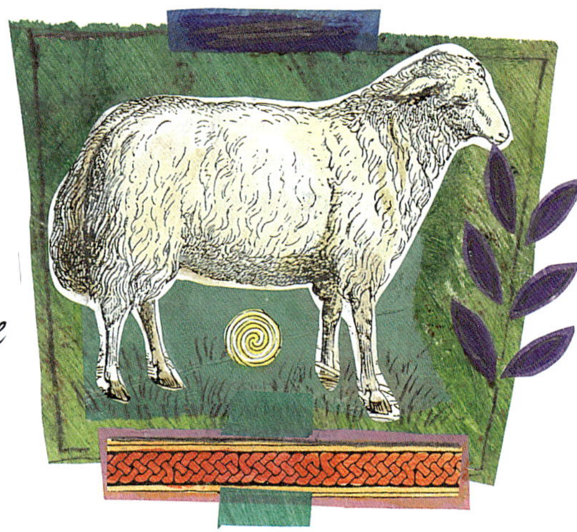

Brigid of Kildare
(c.450–c.523)

Bronach

A traditional Gaelic name, pronounced *BRON-ack*, which comes from the word for 'sorrowful'. It is now used exclusively for girls, although it was once applicable to either sex. The female St. Bronach gave her name to Kilbroney, Co. Down, and her bell is preserved as a relic in the nearby church of Rostrevor.

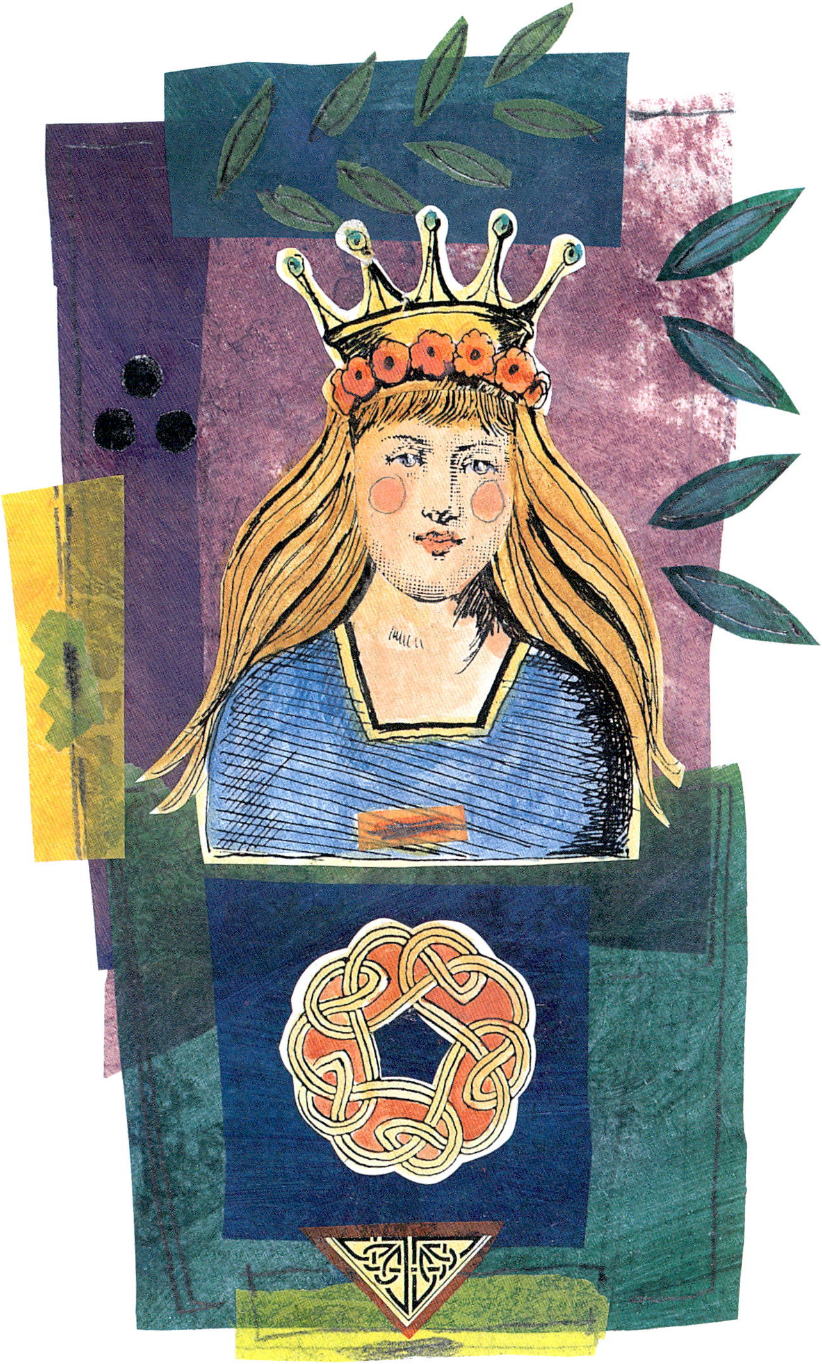

Bridget or Brigid

C

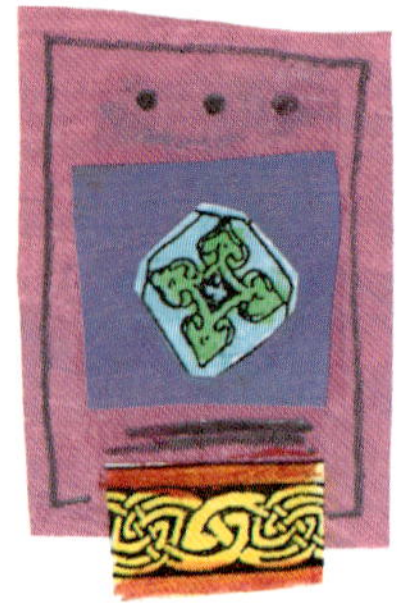

Caitlin, Cathleen

This is an Irish form of Catherine. In Christian lore, a certain Countess Cathleen saved her starving people by offering the devil her soul in exchange for food. Cathleen ni Houlihan (Kathleen O'Hoolihan) is a personification of Ireland, popularized by W.B. Yeats. The Breton form of the name, Katell, is also becoming increasingly common in English-speaking countries.

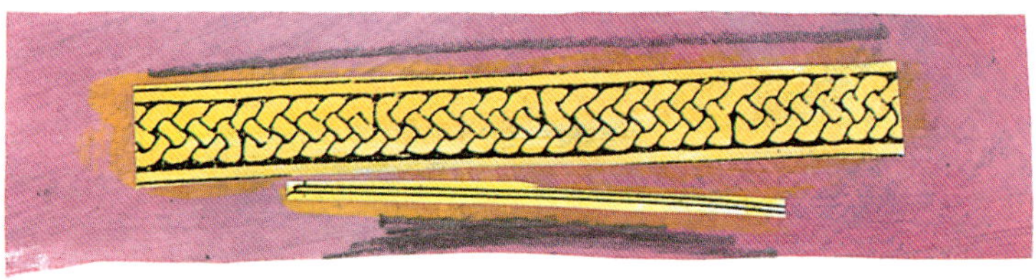

Cathleen ni Houlihan, a personification of Ireland

Caoimhe

This unusual name (pronounced *QUEE-va*) derives from *caomh*, meaning 'comely' or 'beautiful'. It is more commonly found in its male form, Caomhín or Kevin. There is one Irish saint called Caoimhe. Very little is known about her, apart from the fact that her cult was celebrated at Killeavy, Co. Down, and that her feast day is on 2nd November. The name can be anglicized as Keeva.

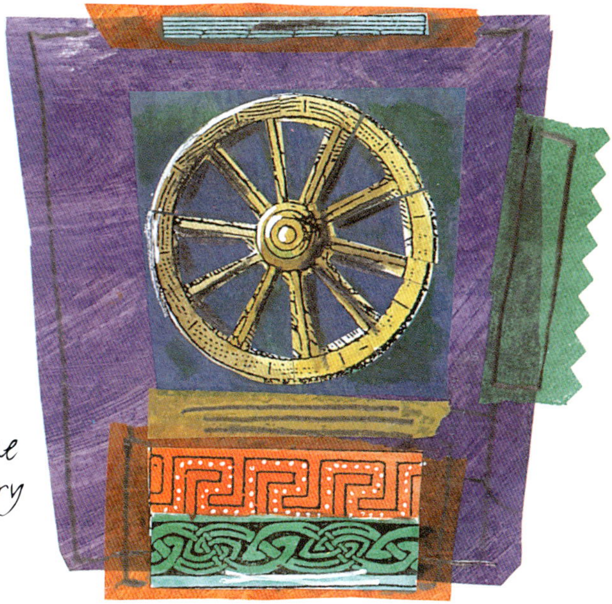

St Catherine (4th century AD)

Catriona

Pronounced *kat-TREE-na*, this name comes from Caterine, an early French form of Catherine, which was introduced into Ireland by the Normans. St. Catherine (4th century AD), whose traditional emblem was a wheel, was very popular in Ireland, and there is a church dedicated to her in Dublin. The Celtic name was made famous by Robert Louis Stevenson's novel *Catriona* (1893).

Ciara, Kira

Meaning 'dark' or 'black', Ciara (pronounced *KEE-ra*) is the feminine form of Ciarán. St. Ciara (d.679) established a religious community at Kilkeary, Co. Tipperary (from *Cill Ciara*, the 'cell' or 'church' of Ciara). This attracted many followers so Ciara persuaded St. Fintan Munnu to help her obtain land for a second convent.

Cliona

Pronounced *KLEE-ONA*, in ancient lore Cliona was the daughter of a druid who served the sea-god, Manannán mac Lir. She lived contentedly in the Land of Promise until her lover lured her away to the land of mortals, where she was drowned by a gigantic wave. In some traditions she is known as the Queen of the Munster fairies because of her habit of stealing young boys away from country fairs.

Clodagh

The origin of the name Clodagh, pronounced *KLOD-ah*, is uncertain, although it seems quite likely that it stems from the river Clóideach in Co. Waterford. In the Celtic world, it was very common for rivers to be called after local goddesses of healing or fertility. Supplicants would attempt to win their assistance by depositing precious objects in the water as a sacrifice to the deity.

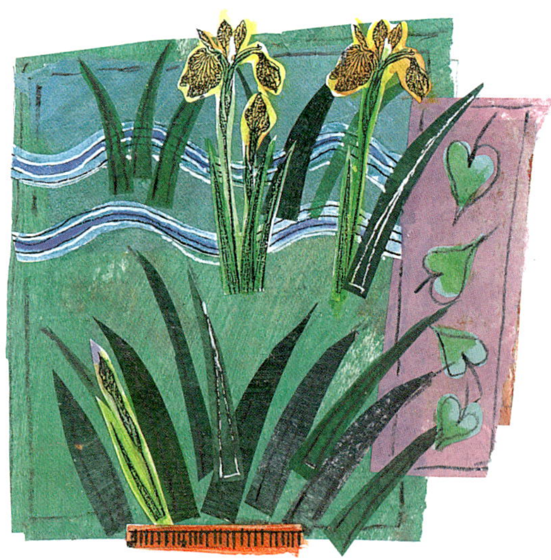

Clodagh

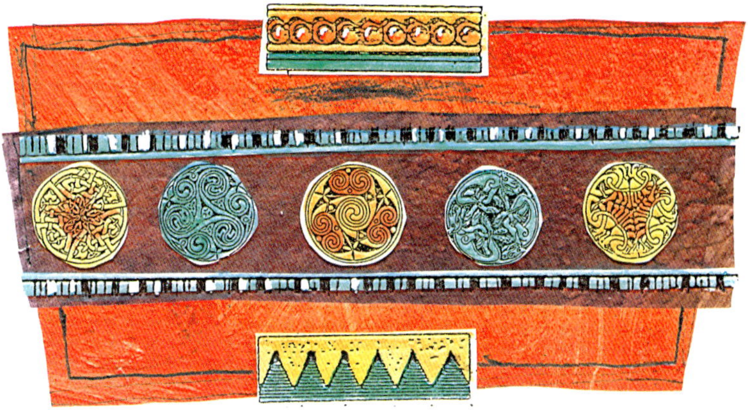

Colette, French novelist (1873–1954)

Colette

This is the feminine, diminutive form of Nicholas, which comes from the Greek for 'victorious people'. The name was introduced into Ireland in the Middle Ages as a result of the popularity of St. Nicholas (4th century AD), the patron saint of children. Internationally, the name is best-known through its association with the French novelist, Colette (1873–1954).

Colleen

This name has entered the English language as a byword for any Irish girl, although ironically it is little used in Ireland itself. It stems from the Gaelic *cailín* ('a girl') and is principally associated with the US and Australia. Examples include the silent-screen actress, Colleen Moore (1901–88) and the Australian novelist, Colleen McCullough, who wrote *The Thorn Birds*.

D

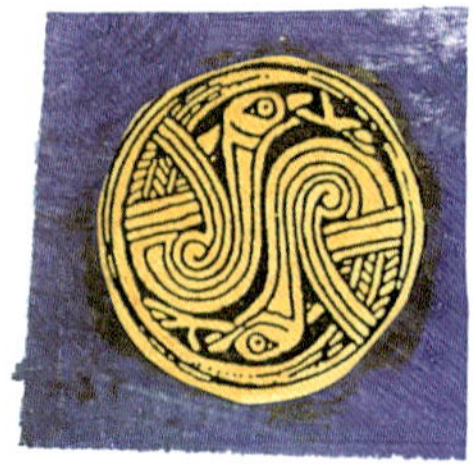

DANA

DANA OR DANU WAS revered as the principal mother-goddess throughout the Celtic world. Among other things, she gave her name to the River Danube. In Ireland there are also strong etymological links with the fertility goddess, Ana. In the US the name was popularized by the actor Dana Andrews (in his case meaning 'a Dane'), while in Europe it is associated with the Irish singer, Dana (born Rosemary Brown).

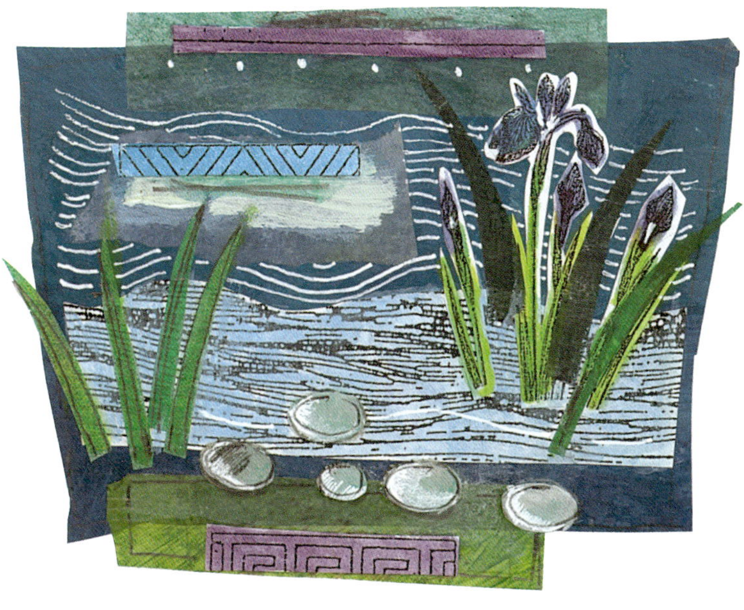

Dana, mother-goddess

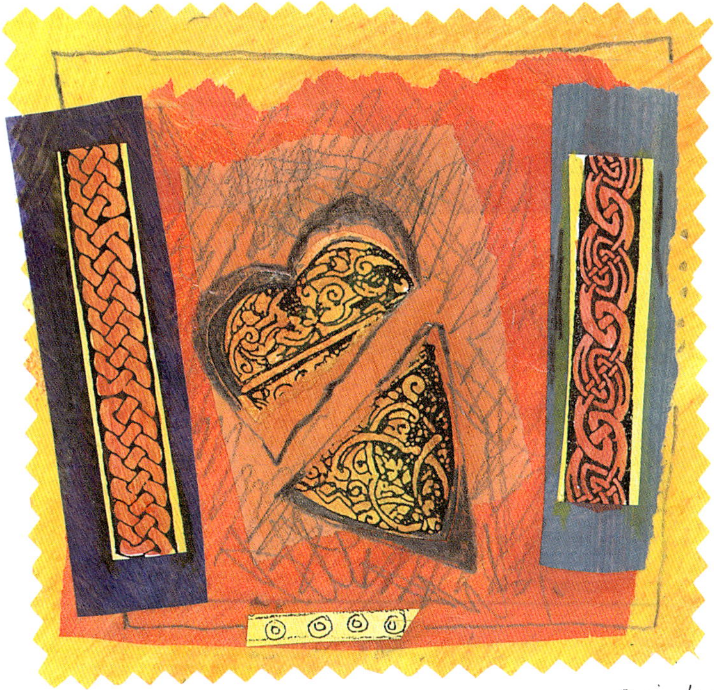

Deirdre, who eloped with Naoise

DEIRDRE

THE NAME OF Deirdre is inextricably linked with one of the most tragic love stories in Irish legend. While still in her mother's womb she cried out, causing Cathbad the druid to predict that she would bring ruin to Ulster. Years later, this prophecy came to pass when Deirdre was betrothed to King Conchobar. Before the wedding, she fell in love with his nephew, Naoise, and the pair eloped. For several years they lived in blissful exile in the Scottish Highlands until they were tricked into returning to Ulster. There, Naoise was treacherously slain and Deirdre hurled herself off Conchobar's chariot, rather than live with the man who had caused her lover's death.

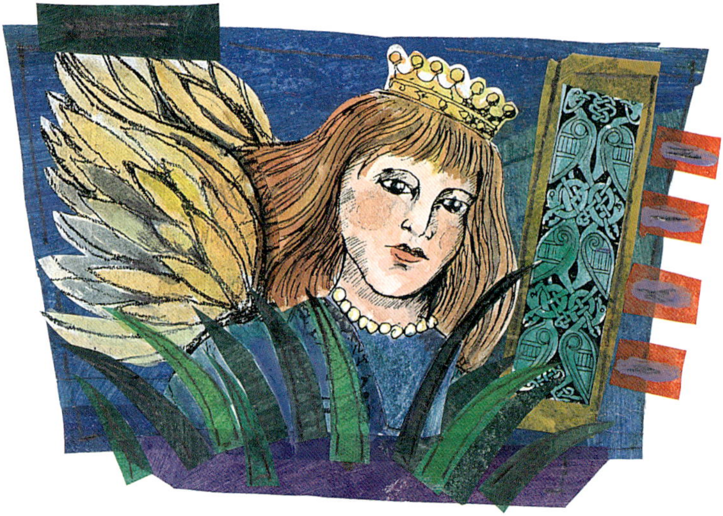

Dervla, daughter of Fál

DERVLA

THIS NAME, PRONOUNCED *DERV-VLA*, is thought to derive from Dearbháil or 'daughter of Fál'. The latter was used as a poetic name for Ireland, because of its associations with a ritual standing stone, located on the mound of Tara. This played a vital part in the inauguration of a new high king, for it was said that the Stone of Fál would cry out, when touched by the rightful heir to the throne.

DERVORGILLA

PRONOUNCED *DERV-OR-GILLA*, this is an anglicized version of Derbforgaill ('daughter of Forgaill'). She was a foreign princess who fell in love with Cú Chulainn and turned herself into a swan to be close to him. In the 12th century, Dervorgilla O'Rourke's adultery sparked off a dispute which prompted the Normans to invade Ireland.

Dorean, Doreen

These are anglicized forms of Doirind or Dáireann. Several characters in Irish mythology shared this name, most notably Doirend, the fairy-woman. She fell in love with Fionn mac Cumhaill and pursued him relentlessly. When he rejected her, she gave him a cup of enchanted mead, which drove him temporarily insane.

Dymphna

Dymphna (pronounced *DYMPH-NA*), is usually said to derive from *damhnait* ('a fawn'). It is chiefly associated with a 7th-century Irish princess who ran away to Flanders to escape the incestuous attentions of her father. He tracked her down and killed her, but miraculous cures occurred near her tomb and she became revered as the patron saint of lunatics and epileptics.

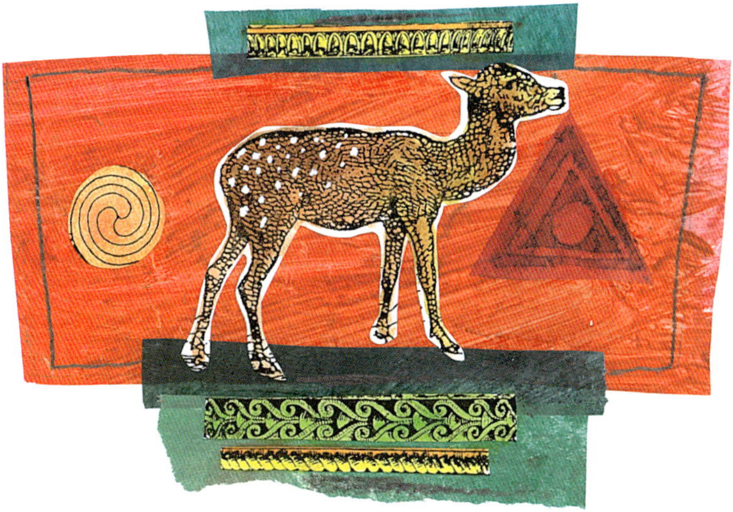

Dymphna, 7th-century Irish princess

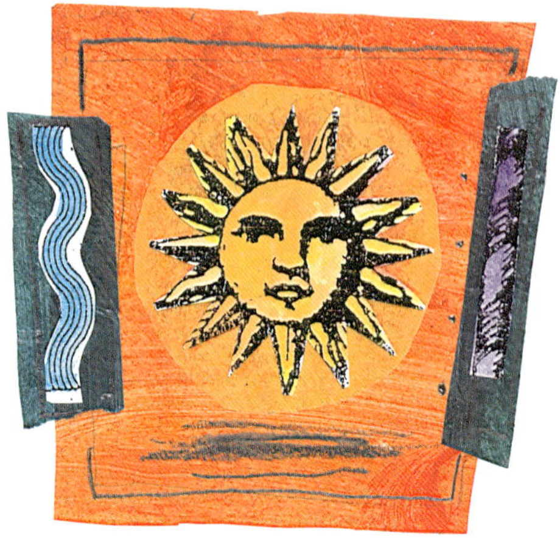

E

Eileen

THIS IS AN ANGLICIZED FORM of Eibhlín, meaning 'light-bearer'. There may also be links with the name Evelyn ('hazelnut'), which was popular with the Normans. Its most famous association is with a love-song, *Eibhlín a rún*, which was composed in the 17th century by the harpist, Cearbhall O'Dálaigh. He used it to persuade his beloved to elope with him.

Emer

EMER (PRONOUNCED *EE-MER*) played a major role in Irish mythology, as the wife of the Ulster hero, Cú Chulainn. The pair were betrothed at the age of seven, but their courtship was long and arduous, since her father opposed the match. Emer was renowned for possessing the 'Six Gifts of Womanhood' (beauty, a gentle voice, sweet words, wisdom, needlework and chastity).

Enya

THIS COMES FROM A Gaelic word for 'kernel' or 'seed'. It is linked with Ainé, the fairy goddess of love and desire. She had many mortal lovers, among them Maurice, Earl of Desmond, who won her by stealing her enchanted cloak. In recent years, the name has become much better known, following the success of the singer Enya (Eithne Ni Bhraonain).

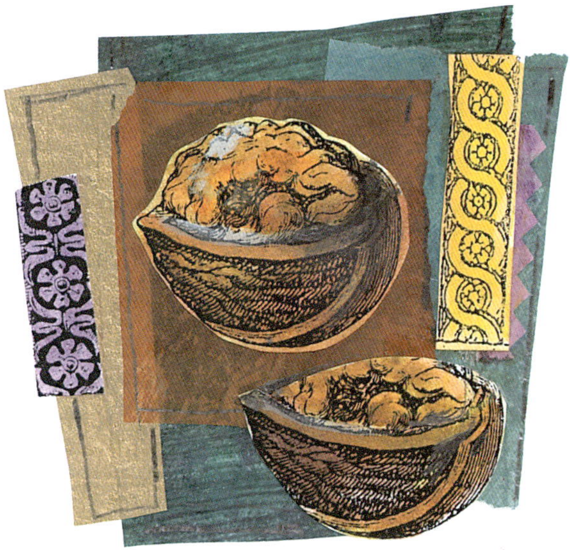

Enya (Eithne Ni Bhraonain)

Erin

ERIN IS A POETIC NAME for Ireland. An ancient text, *The Book of Invasions*, described how three divine sisters – Erin, Banba and Fódla – competed for the honor of giving their name to the country. Erin won the contest with an eloquent speech, calling Ireland 'the fairest land under the sun'. In time, her name evolved into 'Eire'.

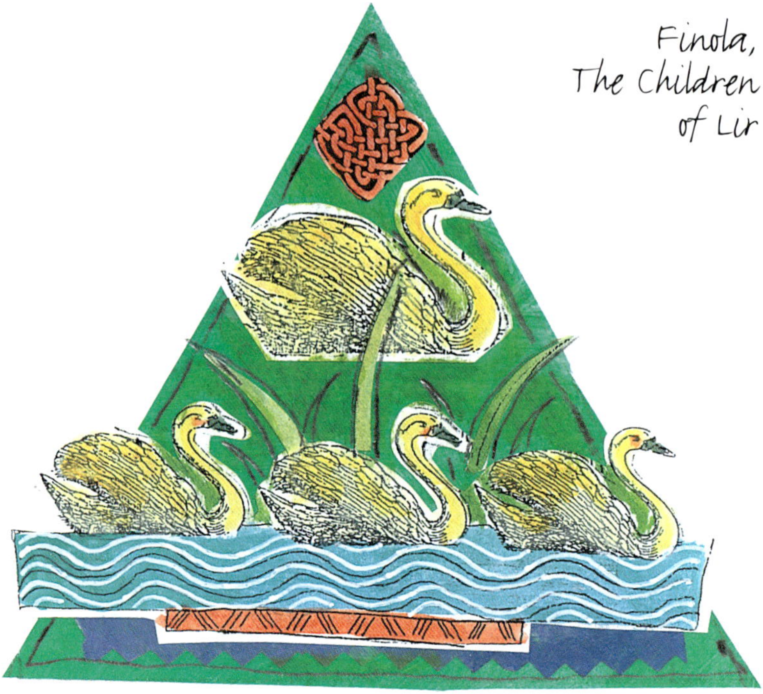

F

FINOLA

THIS IS THE MOST FAMILIAR, modern form of Finnguala, an ancient name meaning 'white shoulders'. It is intimately connected with the famous tale of *The Children of Lir.* In this, Finola and her three brothers were transformed into swans by their jealous stepmother. They remained trapped in this form for 900 years, until a hermit freed them.

G

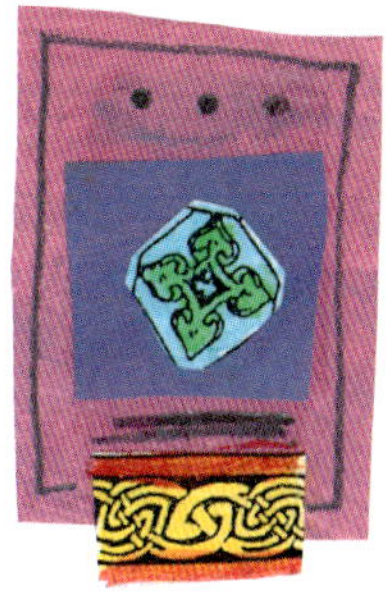

Gráinne, Grania

Pronounced *GRAW-NYA*, this name is irrevocably linked with the greatest love story in Irish legend. Gráinne was destined to be the bride of Fionn mac Cumhaill, but she eloped instead with one of his most noble warriors, Diarmait. For 16 years, the couple fled throughout Ireland, living in forests and caves, until they were rescued by Oenghus, the god of love.

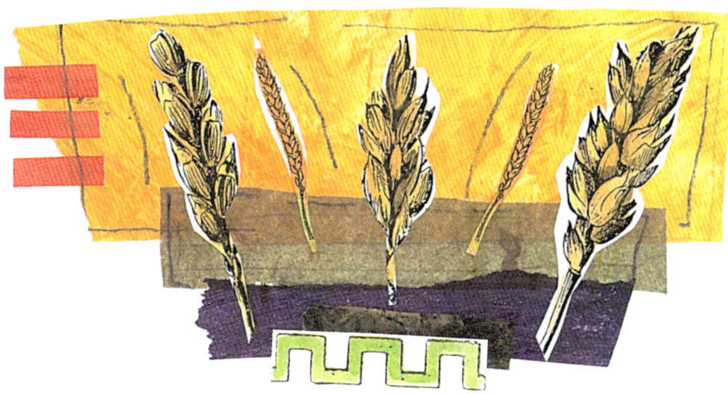

Gráinne

I

Ita, Ida

St. Ita (pronounced *EET-A*) died around 570 and was one of the most famous Irish saints. Known as the 'Foster-mother of the Saints' or the 'White Sun of the Women of Munster', she founded a nunnery at Killeedy (Co. Limerick), where there is a well dedicated to her. In the 19th century, the name featured in a poem by Tennyson (*The Princess*) and an opera by Gilbert and Sullivan (*Princess Ida*).

K

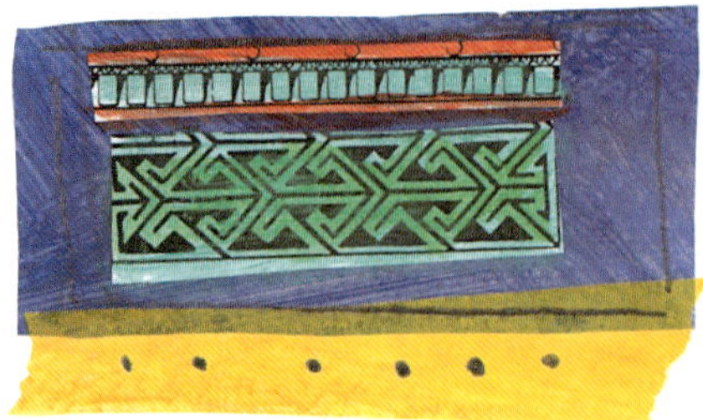

Kayleigh, Kayley

Pronounced *KAY-LEE*, this name stems ultimately from Cáel, a male name deriving from *caol*, the Irish word for 'slender'. As such, it is principally linked with the mythical romance of Cáel and Créd. In recent times, it has been transformed into a popular girl's name, perhaps as an offshoot of Keeley. It gained added publicity when the rock song, *Kayleigh*, became an international hit for Marillion.

Keeley

The source of this name is uncertain. It is likely that it comes from a Gaelic word meaning 'beautiful girl'. Alternatively, it may be a variant of Keelin, which stems from *caol* ('slender') and *fionn* ('fair'), or of the surname Kelly. In the US, it was popularized by the jazz singer, Keely Smith (1932–).

Keelin

This is the anglicized form of Caoilfhinn or Cáelfind, which derive from *caol* ('slender') and *fionn* ('fair'). The name has been associated with a number of minor saints, about whom virtually nothing is known. The principal one, a daughter of Fergus mac Ross, became noted for her piety as a nun. Her biographer noted that 'she won the esteem and affection of her sister nuns by her exactness to every duty, as also by her sweet temper and tender disposition'.

Kelly

In ancient Ireland this name was principally used for boys, although the church of Tallaght recommended it for pre-natal baptisms, since it was applicable to either sex. It derives from *ceallach*, which may mean 'bright-headed' or, more probably, 'a hermit'. For centuries, it was used purely as a surname, but it is now finding favor as a first name for girls.

Kerry

With its ancient hill-forts and beehive huts, County Kerry conjures up a vivid picture of Ireland's romantic past. Small wonder then that so many people have chosen to name their children after it. This trend extends far beyond Ireland and, indeed, the name is especially popular in Australia. It derives from Ciar, the love-child of Fergus mac Roth and Maeve, who is said to have founded the first settlement in Kerry.

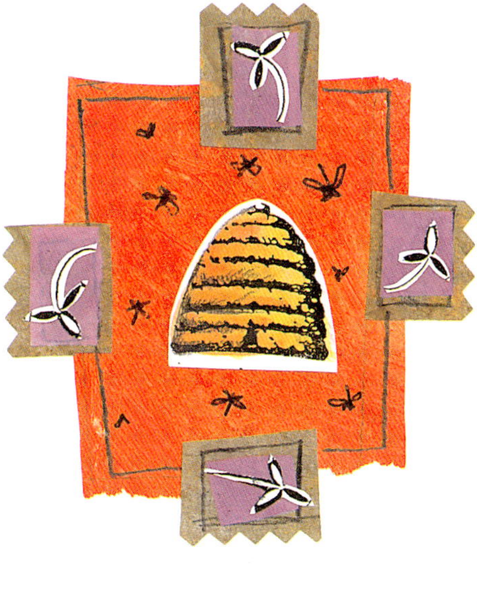

Kerry, love child of Fergus mac Roth and Maeve

L

Liadan

Liadan, ponounced *LEE-DAWN*, means 'gray lady', but it is linked with one of Ireland's most colorful love stories. Liadan fell in love with Cuirithir, but their romance was forbidden because she was a nun. Seeing that it was hopeless, Cuirithir became a monk and set off on a pilgrimage, never to return. Liadan went to his departure point and waited there, gazing out forlornly across the sea, until she died.

M

Maeve

Maeve or Medb was the goddess of sovereignty and a supernatural queen of Connaught. In her role as a goddess, she was central to the inauguration of the high king at Tara. Prospective rulers were expected to 'mate' with her before they could take up office. This ceremony involved libations to the goddess, as her name confirms (its literal meaning is 'she who intoxicates'). In *The Cattle Raid of Cooley*, Maeve was a powerful queen, who led Connaught into a disastrous war against the men of Ulster. During the campaign a squirrel perched on her shoulder, symbolising her ability to shape-shift into any animal form.

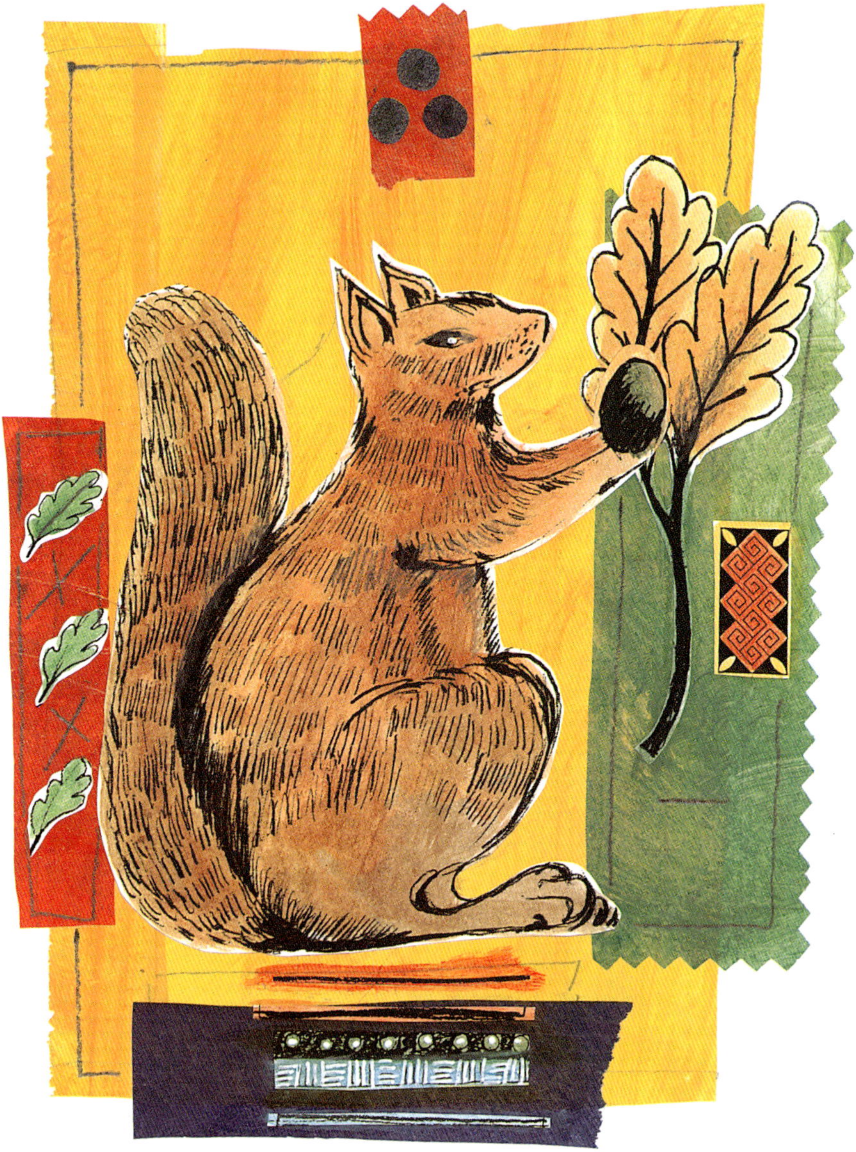

Maeve,
Queen of Connaught

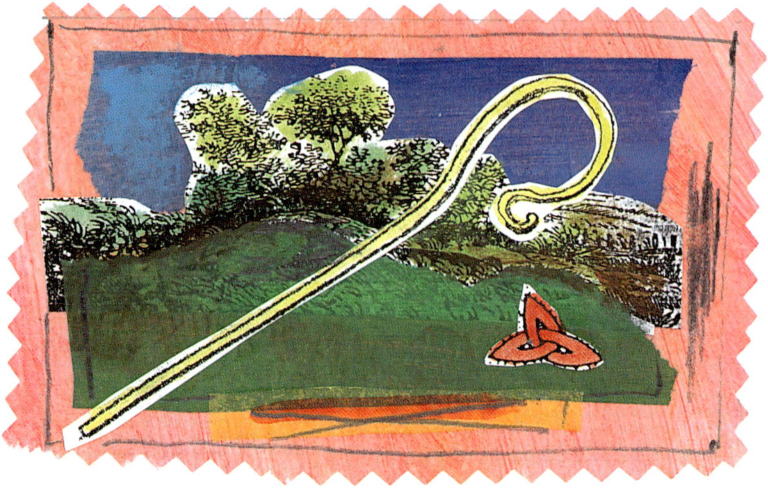

Mairead, Gaelic form of Margaret

MAIREAD

SOMETIMES WRITTEN AS Maighread, Mairead (pronounced *MOY-rade*) is the Gaelic form of Margaret, introduced to Ireland by the Normans. It was widely used during the medieval period, largely due to the popularity of St. Margaret of Antioch. According to tradition, she was the daughter of a pagan priest, who lived as a shepherdess and preached the Gospel, before being beheaded on Diocletian's orders.

MARY, MÁIRE

MARY IS AN ANGLICIZED FORM of the Hebrew name Miriam, which may mean 'sea of bitterness' or 'star of the sea'. With her traditional attribute, the lily of purity, Mary was greatly revered in Ireland, but her name was considered too sacred to use. This situation gradually changed, however, when Muire was reserved for the Virgin, while Máire became acceptable as a personal name.

MAURA

THIS IS WIDELY REGARDED as a variant of Máire, although it may also stem from a Gaelic word for 'dark'. Either way, it became an independent name at a fairly early stage. There was a 5th-century saint named Maura, about whom little is known, apart from the fact that she was martyred with her companion, Britta. The Scottish equivalent of the name is Moira.

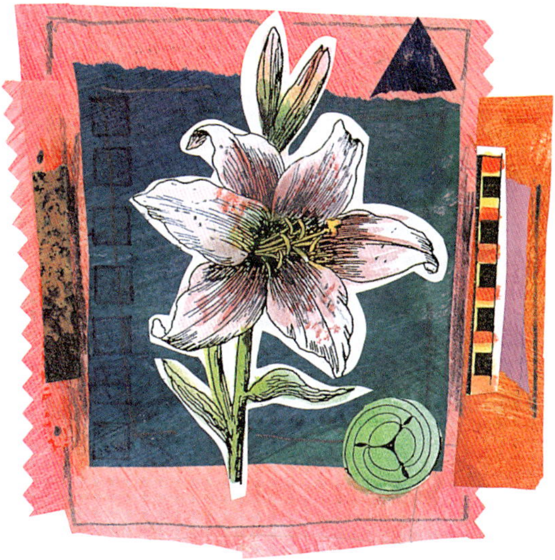

Maura, a 5th-century saint

MAUREEN

THIS COMES FROM THE Gaelic Móirín, which means 'little Mary'. Despite obvious similarities, it is quite separate from Moreen, another popular Irish name, which is a pet form of Mór ('great one'). In modern times, the name has been popularized by the actress Maureen O'Hara, and the tennis-player Maureen Connolly ('Little Mo').

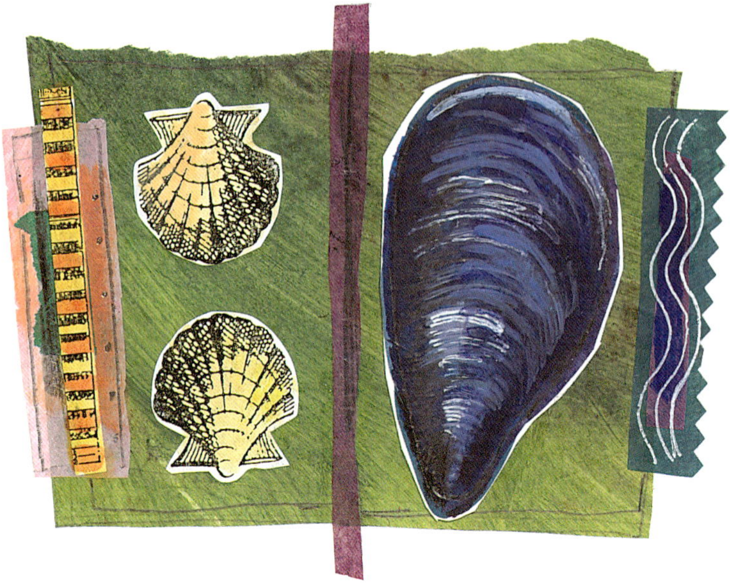

MOLLY

Sweet Molly Malone

MOLLY IS ONE OF the many pet forms of Mary. It is not clear if the name originated in Ireland – some believe that it actually stemmed from the Cornish word, *mailli*. By outsiders, however, it is invariably regarded as an Irish name, largely on the strength of the popular song, *Sweet Molly Malone*. In this, the eponymous heroine wheels her barrow, full of cockles and mussels, through the streets of Dublin.

MORNA, MYRNA

THESE ARE ANGLICIZED FORMS of Muirne, an important figure in Irish mythology. Muirne of the White Neck fell in love with Cumhall, a member of an enemy tribe. Her father, a druid, opposed the match and had Cumhall killed, but not before Muirne had conceived a son. This boy grew up to be Fionn mac Cumhaill, the leader of the Fianna, and he later avenged his father's death.

N

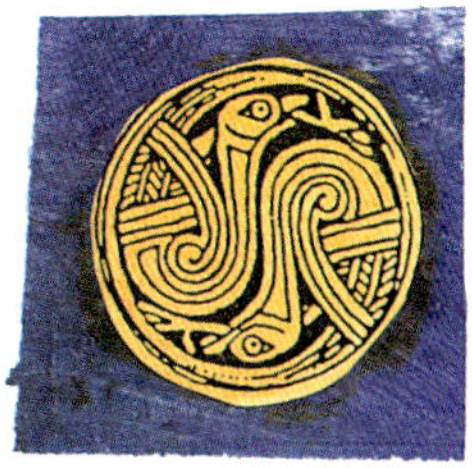

Naomh

Pronounced *KNAVE*, this name comes from *naomh*, which means 'holy' or 'a saint'. It dates back to the early Christian period, when the names for many boys and girls had strong, ecclesiastical overtones. Because of their obvious similarities, Naomh and Niamh are often confused, but there is no direct link between them.

Nessa

In Irish legend, Nessa was the daughter of Eochaidh Sálbuidhe and the mother of Conchobar, the Ulster king featured in *The Cattle Raid of Cooley*. Her first husband was a royal giant named Fachtna Fáthach, but he was not the father of her child. This was Cathbad the Druid, who had won Nessa by answering her riddle, 'what is the hour lucky for?', with the reply, 'begetting a king upon a queen'. This prophecy was fulfilled when Nessa tricked her second husband, Fergus, into giving up his throne, so that Conchobar could rule in his place.

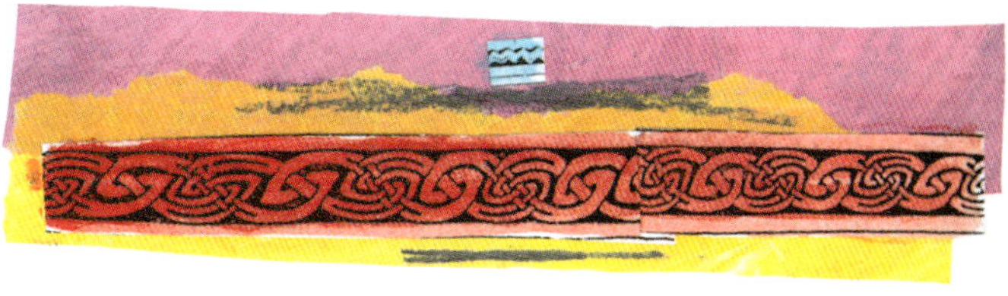

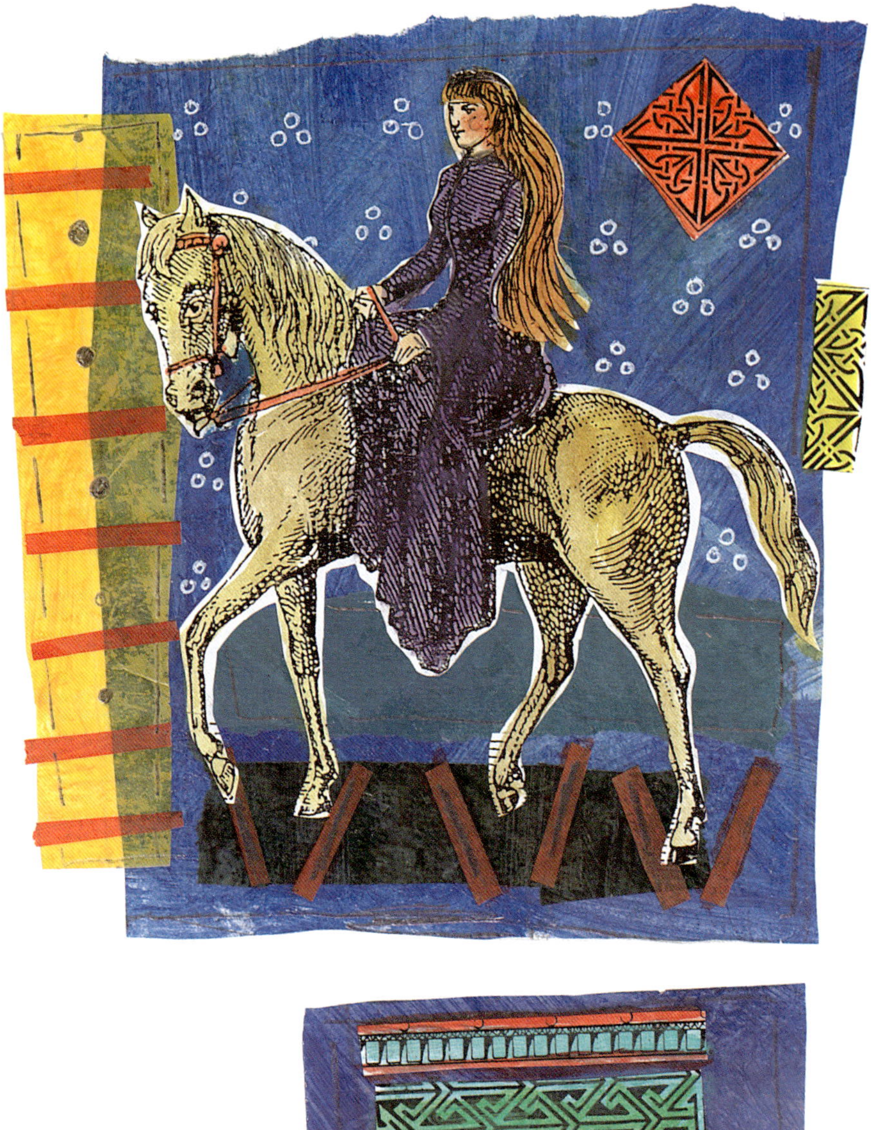

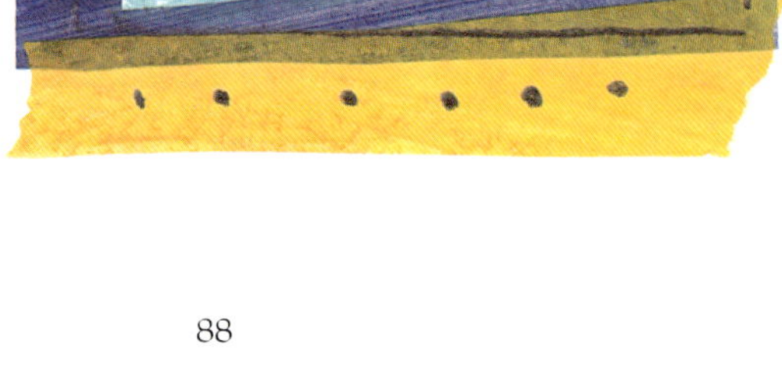

Niamh of the Golden Hair

NIAMH

MEANING 'RADIANCE' OR 'brightness', this name (pronounced *KNEE-ov*) is closely bound up with the Oisin legend. One day, Niamh of the Golden Hair rode up to the warrior and invited him to join her. Entranced, Oisin climbed up behind Niamh and they rode off to Tir na nOg (the Land of Youth), where they lived contentedly for 300 years. Oisin then revisited his homeland but, on dismounting from Niamh's horse, he aged dramatically and could no longer return to her.

Nola, derived from the Latin for 'bell'

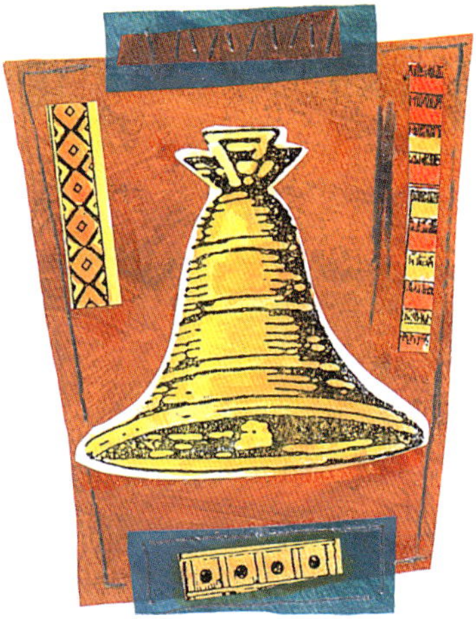

NOLA

THERE IS SOME DISPUTE about the origin of this name. It is usually regarded as a diminutive form of Finola or Finnguala ('white shoulders'). As such, it is also linked with Nuala, which has now become a separate name. Alternatively, it may be a feminine form of Nolan ('chariot-fighter') or derive from the Latin for 'bell' (so-called because church-bells were said to have been invented in the Italian town of Nola).

Nora

Nora is sometimes regarded as a shortened form of Eleanor ('a torch'), but it is more likely to derive from Honora. This was a Latin name, meaning 'honor', which became extremely popular in Ireland during the Middle Ages. It is closely associated with the O'Brien family, the descendants of Brian Boru.

Nora, a shortened form of Eleanor

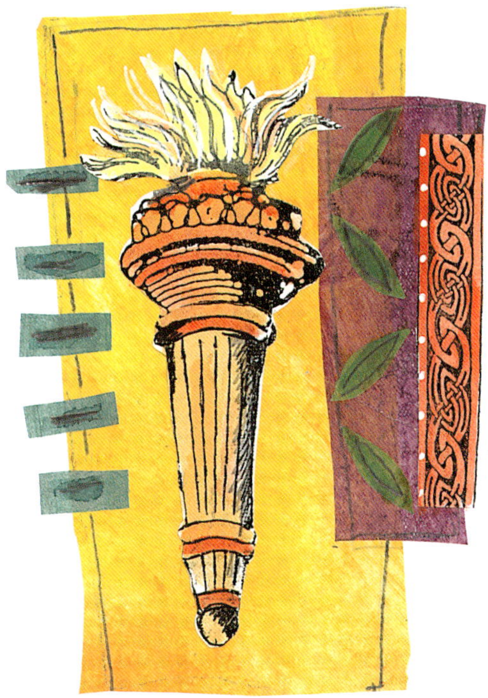

Noreen

Noreen is one of a number of names which developed as variants of Honora. Its immediate source is the Gaelic Noírín, which is a diminutive of Nora, but it can also be linked with names such as Onorina, Norine and Nureen. Onorina Brenach (d.1552) was the Baroness of Courtstown.

O

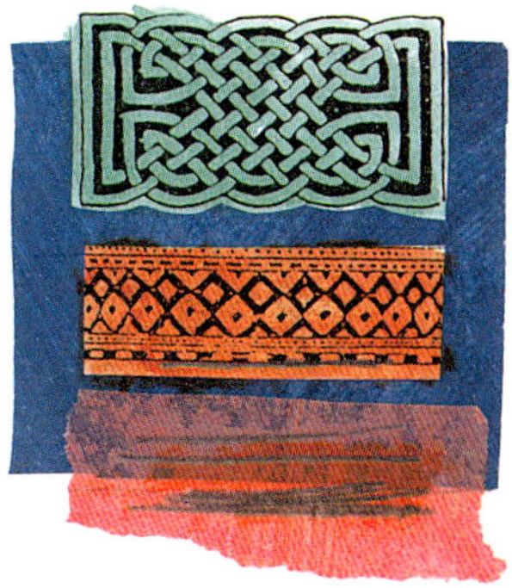

OONA, OONAGH

THIS IS A VARIANT OF Una, which probably derives from *uan* ('a lamb'). In Irish legend, the name is mainly associated with Una, Queen of the Fairies, who had long golden hair, which reached to the ground. Another Una gained fame through her son, Conn of the Hundred Battles, who became the first King of Tara.

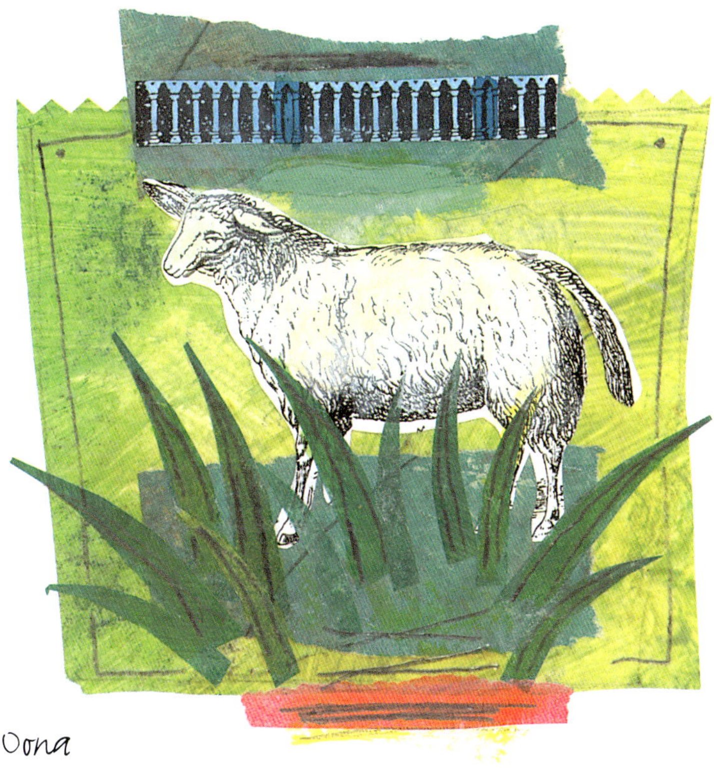

Oona

ORLA

THE LITERAL MEANING of this name is 'golden princess'. It was extremely popular in pre-Norman Ireland – in a 12th-century list of famous women, prepared by an anonymous chronicler in Fermanagh, it ranked fifth in terms of numbers. Brian Boru (d.1014), the most famous of the high kings, had both a sister and a niece called Orlaith.

P

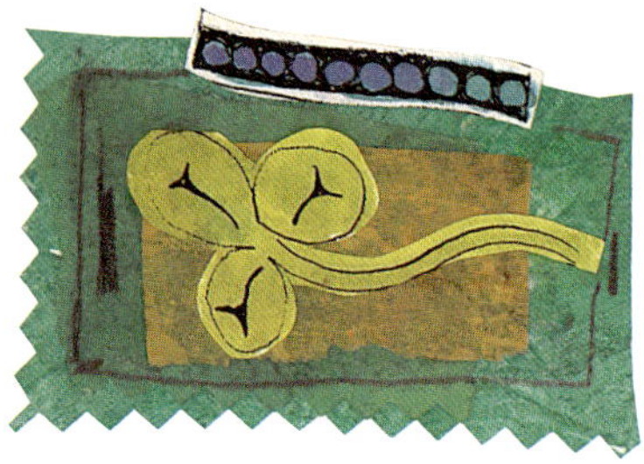

PATRICIA

MEANING 'NOBLE', Patricia is the feminine form of Patrick. Its origins are Latin, as St. Patrick himself came from a Romano-British family. The name has obvious relevance to Ireland, but in fact it is less common there than some of its variants. These include Pat, Patsy, Paití, Trish and Trisha.

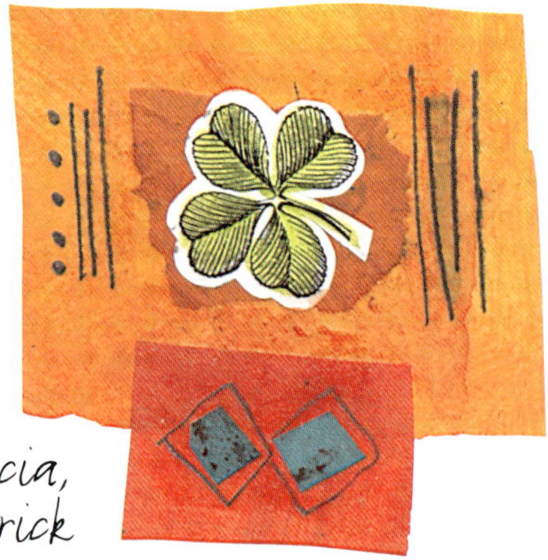

Patricia, feminine form of Patrick

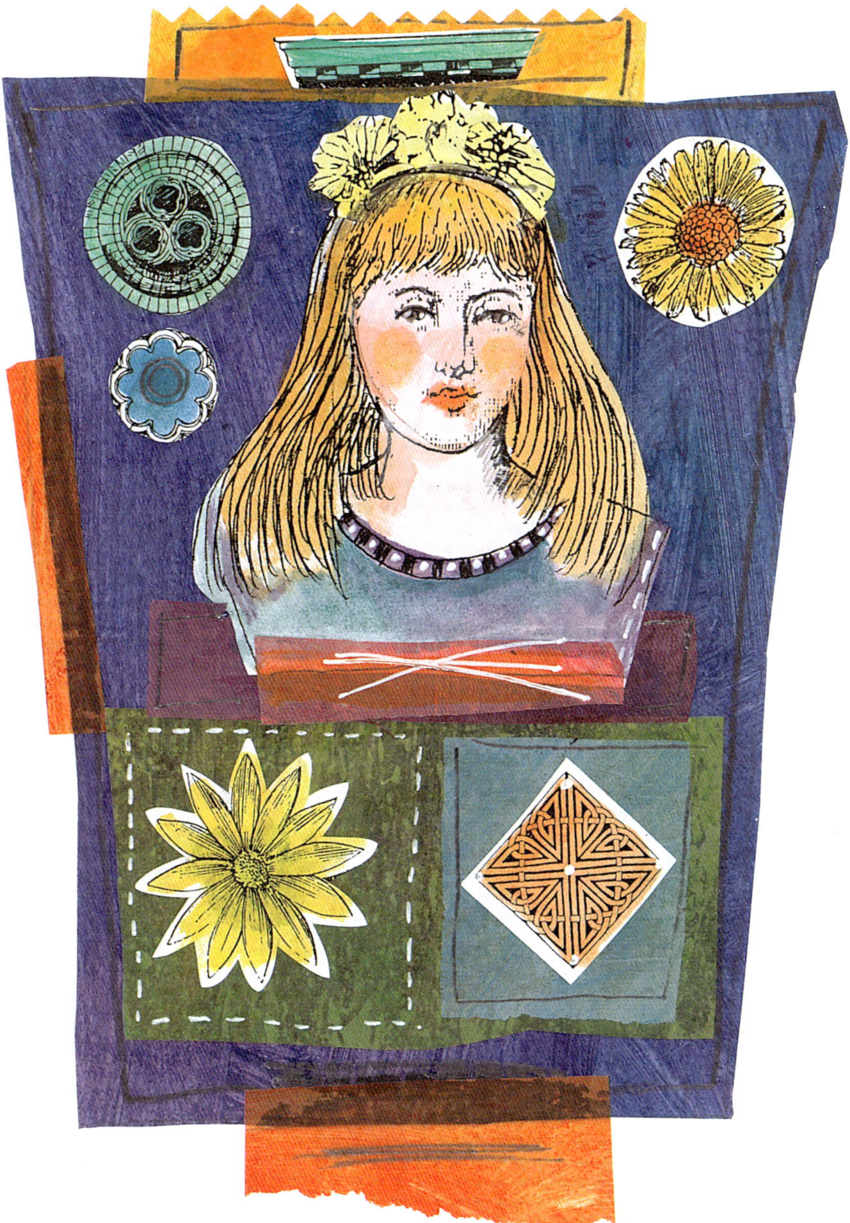

Orla, 'golden princess'

R

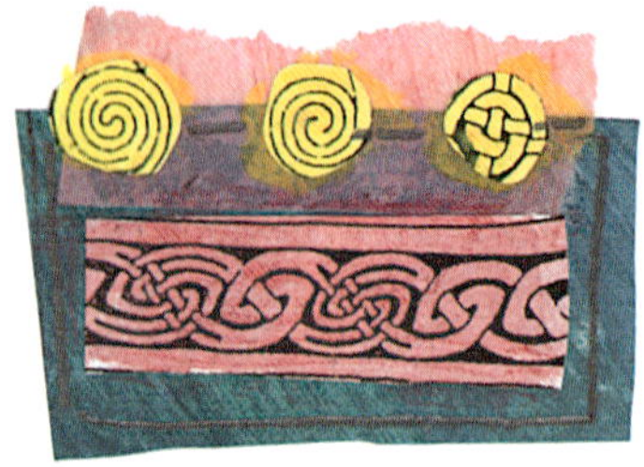

Regan

As a girl's name, this may well have originated with Shakespeare's *King Lear* (1605). In the play, Regan is one of the king's ungrateful daughters, who throws him out of her home in the middle of a raging storm. The name Rígán ('kingly'), however, had long been established as a boy's name in Ireland. In time, this became more common as the surname, Reagan.

Rionach

Although Rionach (pronounced *REEN-uch*) is sometimes regarded as a shortened form of Catriona, it is a traditional Gaelic name, meaning 'queenly'. In Irish lore, Rionach was the wife of one of the first high kings, Niall of the Nine Hostages, and the ancestor of many important Irish dynasties. The name was also borne by two Irish saints, whose feast days are celebrated on 18th December and 9th February.

Róisín

Pronounced *ROE-ISH-EEN*, this name means 'little rose'. Its roots are Latin and it was introduced into Ireland by the Normans. The name is chiefly associated with a 16th- or 17th-century poem called *Róisín Dubh* ('Dark Little Rose'), which is attributed to Owen Roe MacWard. Its eponymous heroine is usually regarded as a personification of Ireland.

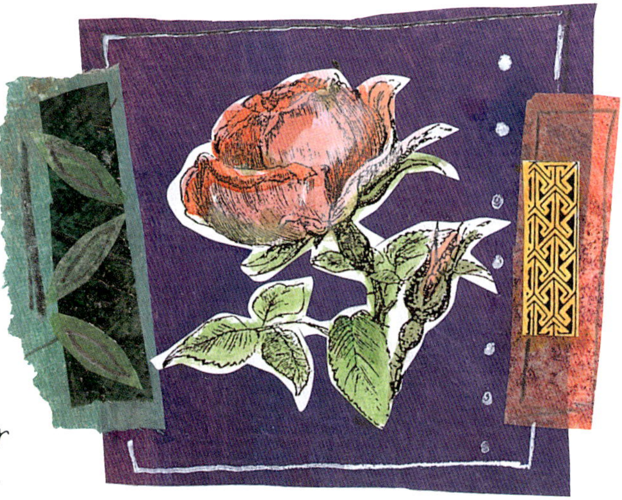

Róisín or Rosaleen

Rosaleen

This is an anglicized form of Roisin, which has now become generally accepted as a separate name. Its popularity stems from *Dark Rosaleen*, the title which James Clarence Mangan gave to his translation of *Róisín Dubh* (1847). Both names carry the same patriotic overtones.

Rowan

Originally used as a name for both boys and girls, this name reflects the importance of the rowan tree in early Irish myth. Rowan-berries were thought to offer protection against fairy spells and to stimulate rejuvenation. Irish druids regarded the rowan as more sacred than the oak, using it as one of the symbols in their ogham alphabet. In later, Christianized myths rowan twigs were wielded as magic wands by malevolent druids.

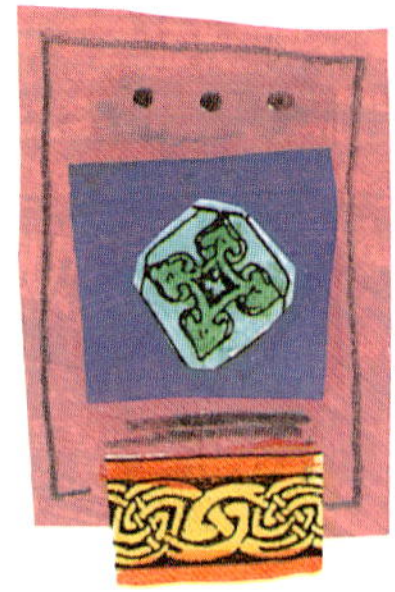

S

Sadbh

Pronounced *SYVE*, this was a very popular name in the Middle Ages. It derives from the tale of Sadb, a gentle fawn, who was transformed into a beautiful woman and became Fionn's bride. Their romance did not last long, however, for an evil druid turned bv her back into a deer. Fionn hunted for her for seven years, but their paths never crossed again.

Saoirse

This is a relatively modern name, pronounced *SEER-sha*, which means 'freedom'. It came into use in the 1920s and, not surprisingly, has strong, patriotic overtones. It was particularly popular during the period of the Irish Free State, which came into being in 1922 and survived until 1937, when its name was changed to Eire.

Shannon

This name, which is mainly popular in the US, is borrowed from Ireland's longest river. In its turn, this derives from the river's tutelary goddess, Sinann. She was a granddaughter of the sea-god Lir and, in a quest for knowledge, she visited Connla's well, which was the fount of all wisdom in Ireland. When she attempted drink from its waters, however, the spirit of the spring was enraged by at her presumption, however, the waters of the spring gushed out and drowned her.

Sheena

This is an English form of Siné, which is popular both in Ireland and Scotland. Its origins are not entirely clear, but it seems likely that it is simply an Irish version of Jane ('God is gracious'). It may also be a shortened form of Sinead. The name gained a higher profile, following the success of the singer, Sheena Easton.

Sheila

Sheila is an anglicized spelling of Síle, which in turn was probably borrowed from the Latin name, Cecilia. Despite its Gaelic roots, the name is more widely used outside Ireland, and a 'Sheila' has become a slang term for an Australian woman. In 1471, Síle O'Neill mounted a famous defence of Omagh Castle, in the absence of her husband. A sheela-na-gig was a fertility carving, frequently found in medieval Ireland.

Sinead

Pronounced *shin-aid*, this stems from Jehanne or Jeannette, both of which were introduced by the Normans. Its English form is Janet. The name has been popularized by Sinead Flanagan (1878–1975), the writer who became the wife of Eamon de Valera; by the actress Sinead Cusack; and by the maverick rock star, Sinead O'Connor.

SIOBHAN

THIS IS THE IRISH form of Joan, pronounced *shiv-AWN*. It derived originally from the Anglo-Norman name Jehanne ('God is gracious') and was much favored by the mistresses of the invaders' newly-built castles. The name can be found in a growing number of different spellings, such as Shevaun and Chevonne. It has become increasingly popular in recent years, thanks to such figures as Siobhan Davies (dancer and choreographer), Siobhan Fahey (rock musician) and, above all, the actress Siobhan McKenna (1923–86). A native of Belfast, she enjoyed great success at the Abbey Theatre in Dublin, as well as in films and television.

Siobhan,
Irish form of Joan

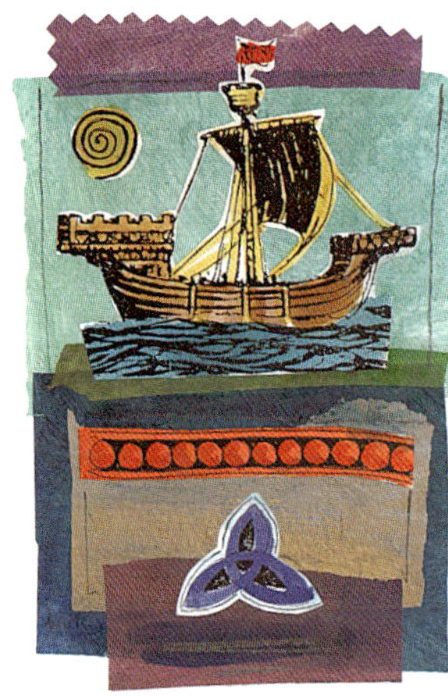

SORCHA

PRONOUNCED *SURK-HA*, this comes from a Gaelic word meaning 'brightness' or 'radiance'. It is sometimes regarded as an Irish form of Sarah, but there is no evidence to support this. The name was extremely popular in the Middle Ages, but then entered a decline. It has enjoyed a revival in recent years, partly due to figures such as the actress, Sorcha Cusack.

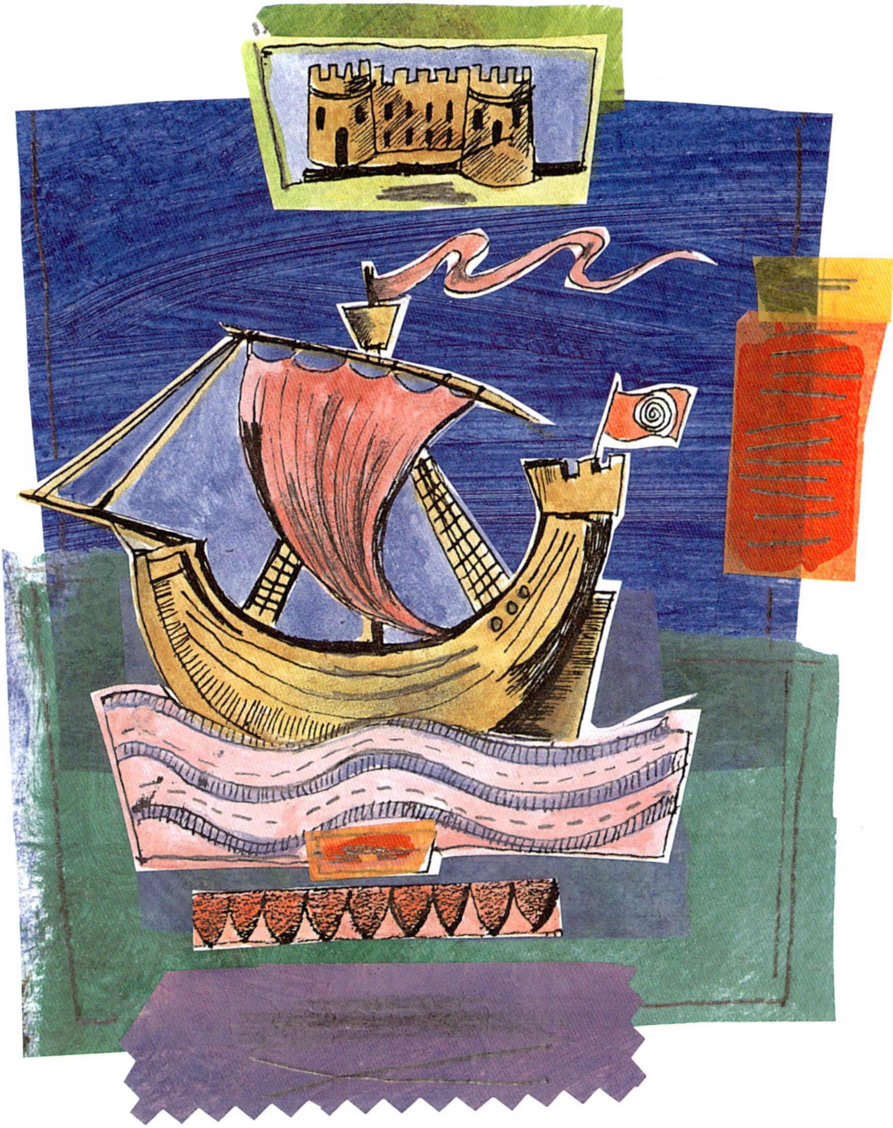

Siobhan McKenna (1923–86)

The Tara brooch

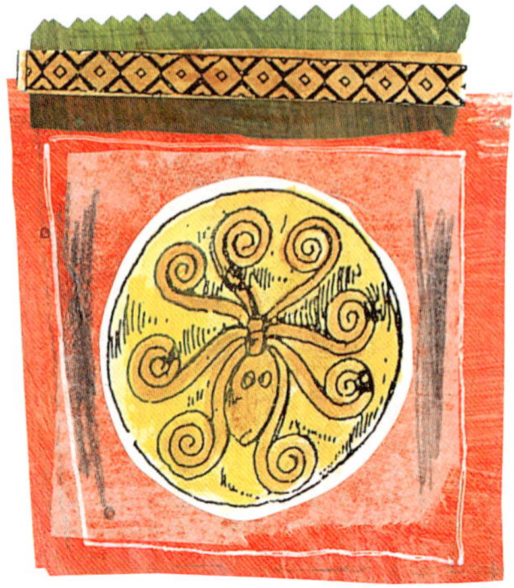

T

Tara

Perhaps the most evocative of all Irish names, Tara is derived from a prehistoric burial site in Co. Meath. From ancient times, this was revered as a place of great importance. It was the site where the high kings were chosen and initiated, as well as the spot where St. Patrick converted his pagan enemies. The Tara Brooch, one of Ireland's greatest Celtic treasures, was named after it and, in 1807, Tom Moore wrote a famous ballad about 'Tara's Halls'.

Teresa

This is an imported name, which probably derives from the Greek word for 'reaper'. It gained great popularity in Ireland, because people wanted to name their children after St. Teresa of Avila (1515–82). She reformed the Carmelite Order and became the first woman to be accepted as a Doctor of the Church. More recently, the name's reputation has been enhanced by the work of Mother Teresa (1910–97).

Saints' Feast Days

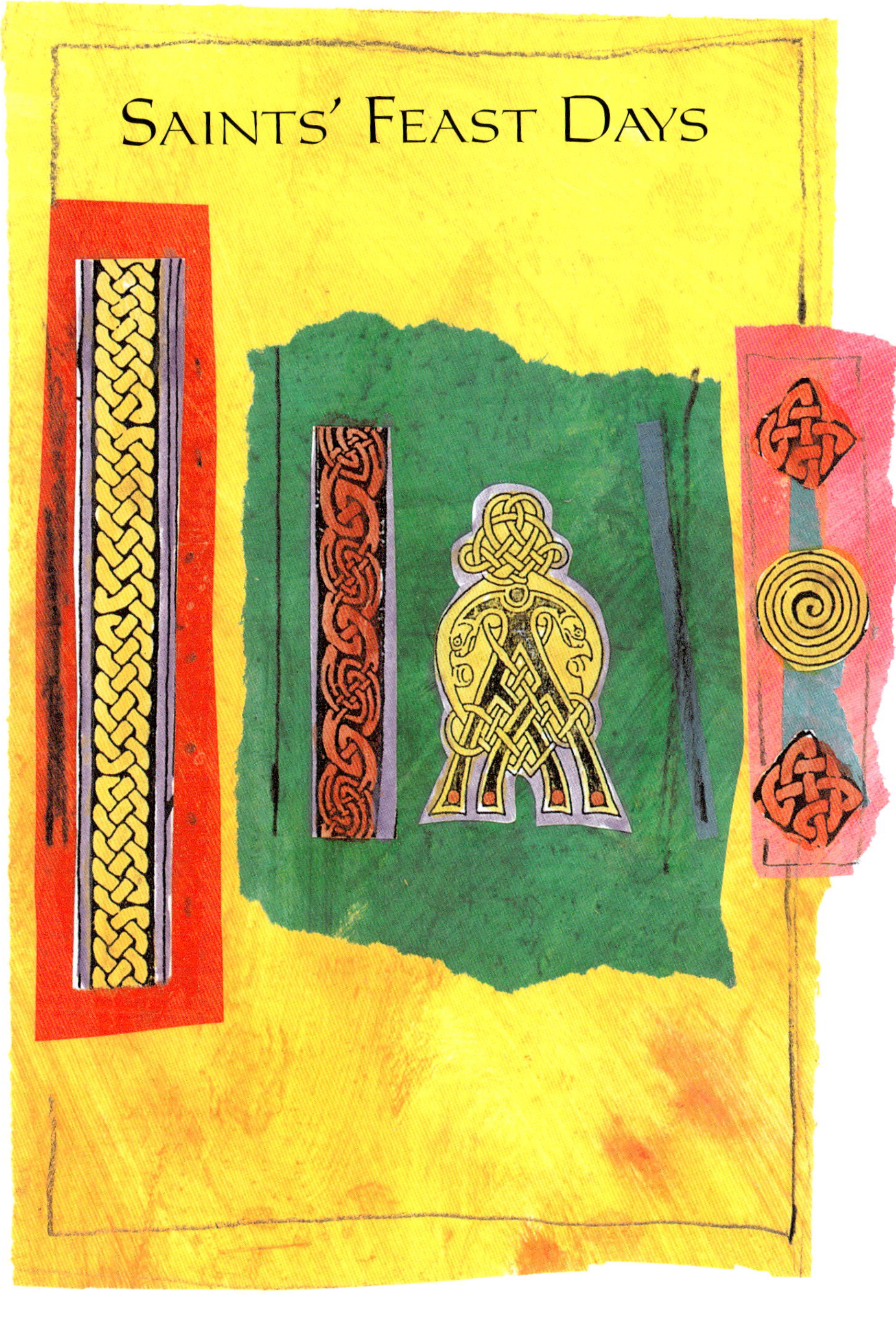

SAINTS' FEAST DAYS

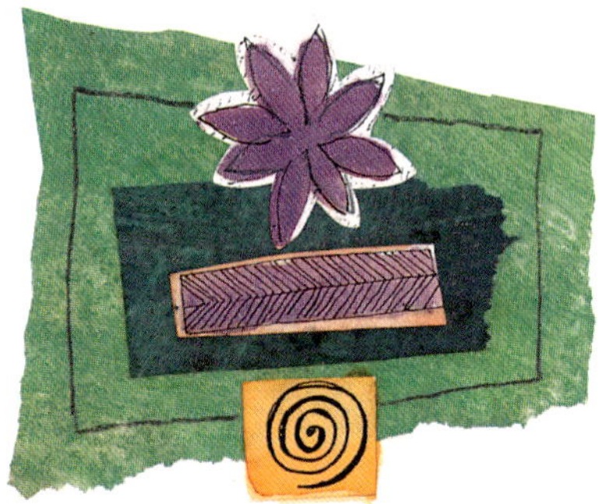

UNTIL RECENTLY, it was quite common for parents to name their child after one of the saints whose feast day coincided with the date of birth of their new arrival.

The veneration of saints dates back to the 2nd century. Initially, the term was restricted to martyrs, who had given their lives for their faith. On the anniversary of their death, followers would gather at the grave to honor the martyr. From the outset, the emphasis was on rejoicing in the sacrifice, rather than mourning for the individual. As Christianity spread, these feast days were no longer local affairs, but were acknowledged by the entire Church.

Gradually, as the persecution of Christians became less common, the definition of sainthood changed. The term was no longer applied solely to martyrs, but could also refer to those who had made a significant contribution to the Church. These saints were known as 'Confessors'. Most of the Irish saints fall into this very broad category, since they were revered for their part in bringing Christianity to the island. In general, they were either the missionaries who founded the first churches, the abbots who

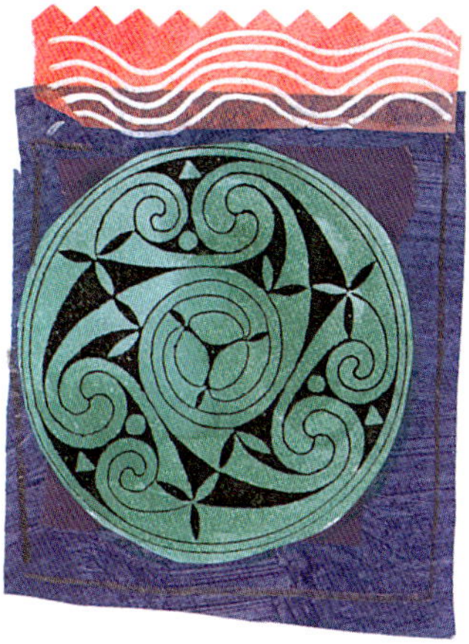

ran the great monastic houses, or the hermits who demonstrated their piety by becoming 'exiles for Christ'.

As the number of saints proliferated, with nearly every day becoming the feast of one or more saints, the Papacy began to regulate the process of canonization to ensure that candidates measured up to their high standards. Although some Irish saints were not recognized by the Pope, as their cult was too local or too poorly documented, they played an important role in Ireland's early history and many of their names – listed on the following pages with girls in italics – are still in use today.

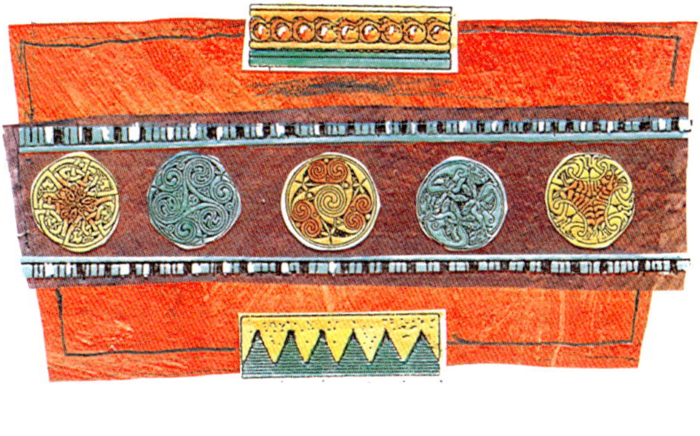

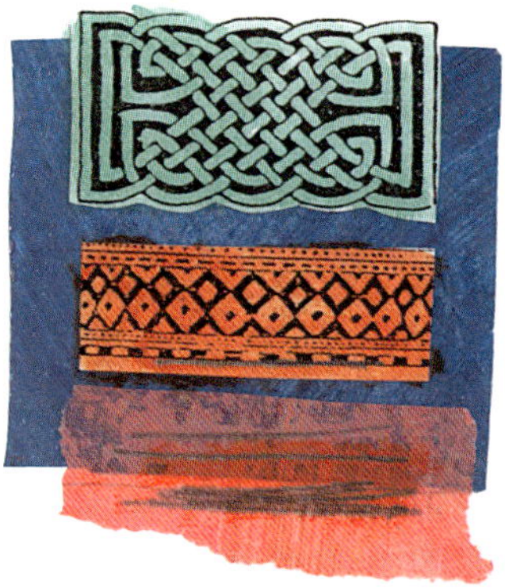

January

1st. **Mary, Mother of God**
Oisin, *Fainche*
2nd. Mainchín
3rd. Killian
4th. Aodh
5th. Ciarán
6th. Dermot
7th. Donnan, Eimhín
8th. Finan
9th. Faolan, Brendan
10th. Dermot
11th. Ronan, Suibhne
12th. Conan, Cumin
13th. Colman, Ronan
14th. Flann
15th. *Aithche*
16th. Dermot, Maelíosa
17th. Ernan, Ultan
19th. Fachtna, Suibhne

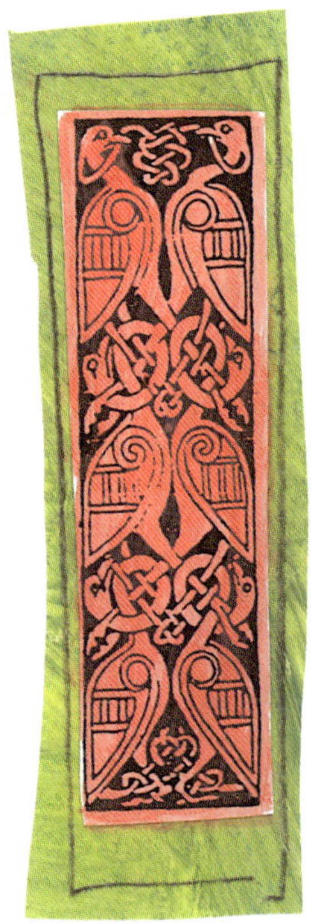

FECHIN (c.580/90–665) FEAST DAY 20TH JAN.

THIS IS THE BEST-KNOWN of the five Irish saints called Fechin, pronounced *FECK-in*, which probably derives from *fiach* ('a raven'). He was born at Bile Fechin (Co. Sligo) and trained at Achonry by St. Nathy. Fechin founded several monasteries, the largest at Fore (Co. Westmeath). During the saint's lifetime, this was home to more than 300 monks. Fechin died of the yellow plague in 665, but his followers spread his cult in Scotland, where his name is preserved in Ecclefechan (from the ecclesia or 'church' of Fechin) and St. Vigean.

20TH. AONGHUS, FERGUS, FECHIN
21ST. FLANN, FAINCHE
22ND. LONAN
23RD. LUCAN, *CANICE*
25TH. AODH
26TH. ERNIN
27TH. LUCAN
28TH. MELLAN
29TH. CRONAN, *BLÁTH*
30TH. ENAN, *AILBE*
31ST. AIDAN, *CANICE*

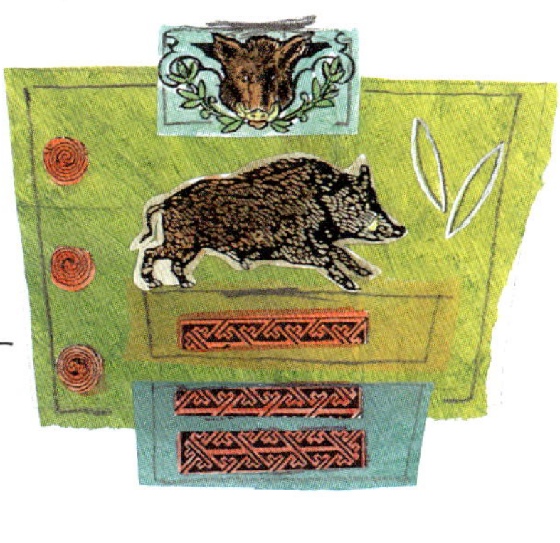

Dermot, or Diarmait – feast day, 16th January

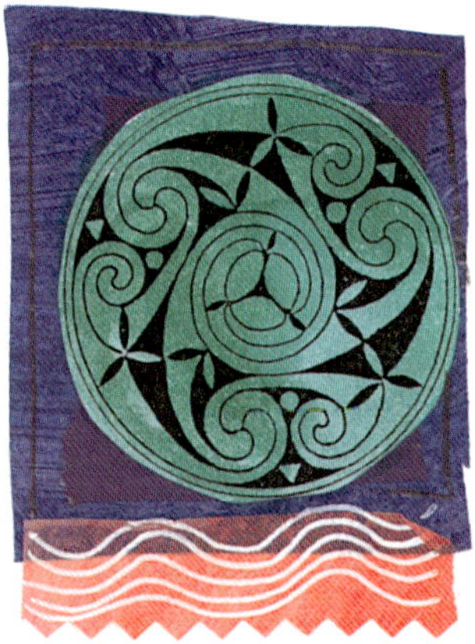

February

Loman (5th century?)

feast day 4th Feb.

An ancient tradition records that Loman was a nephew of St. Patrick, and that he accompanied the saint on his mission to Ireland. While Patrick went to confront King Laoghaire at Tara, Loman took their boat up the Boyne. On his travels, he managed to convert Fechtern, the Lord of Trim (Co. Meath), who appointed him as the region's first bishop. More reliable sources suggest that St. Loman may actually have held this post at a much later date, probably in the 7th century.

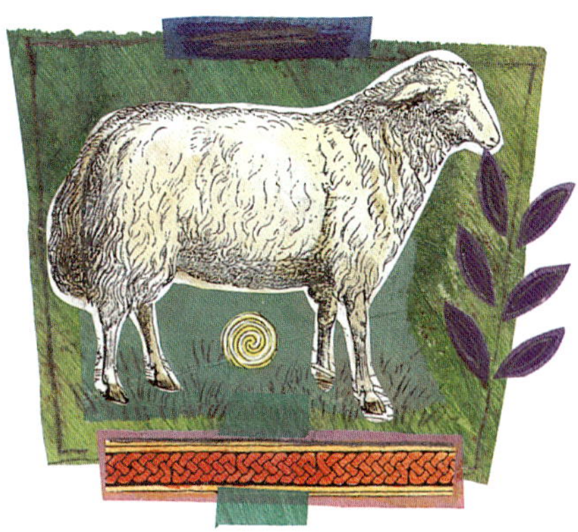

Bridget, or Brigid – feast day, 1st February

1st. *Brigid*
2nd. Colman
3rd. *Keelin*
4th. Ciarán, Loman
5th. Finghin
6th. Colm
7th. Mellan, Aodh, Loman, Lonan
8th. Fiachra, Fáilbhe
9th. Ronan, *Rionach*
10th. Cronan
11th. Finnian, *Gobnait*
12th. Aloysius, Siadhal
13th. Conan, Finan
14th. Mainchín, Caomhán
15th. Fergus, Bearach
16th. Aonghus, Aodh
17th. Cormac, Fintan
18th. Colman, Aonghus
19th. Odran, Fechin
20th. Cronan
21st. Colman, Fintan
22nd. Caomhán
23rd. Ernin
24th. Ciarán, Cumin
25th. Cianán
26th. Beacan, *Eithne*
27th. Comhghan
28th. Ernin

March

1st. Colm, Seanán
2nd. Cuan, Finnian, Conall
3rd. Killian, Fachtna
5th. Carthach, Ciarán
6th. Cairbre, Odran, *Brigid*
8th. Conan, Cronan, Siadhal
9th. Aloysius, Proinnséas, Séadna, *Brigid*
10th. Colman, Fáilbhe
11th. Aonghus
12th. Killian
13th. Caomhán
14th. Ultan, Flannán
15th. Eoghan
16th. Aidan, Finan, Abban
17th. Patrick, Beacan, Tierney
18th. Coman, Caomhán, Conall
20th. Conan, Aidan
21st. Enda
22nd. Fáilbhe

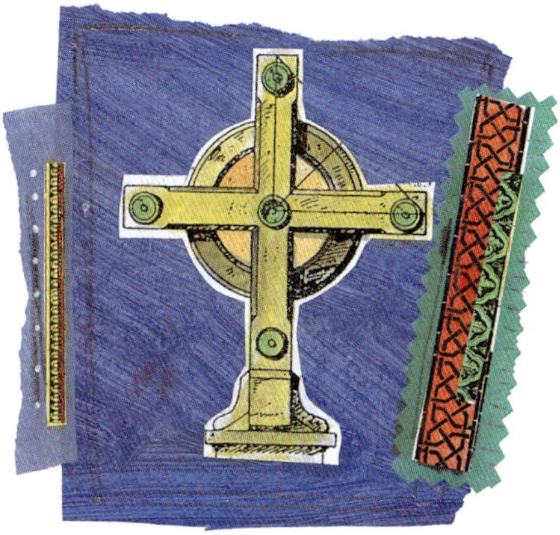

Ciarán, or Kieran – feast day, 5th March

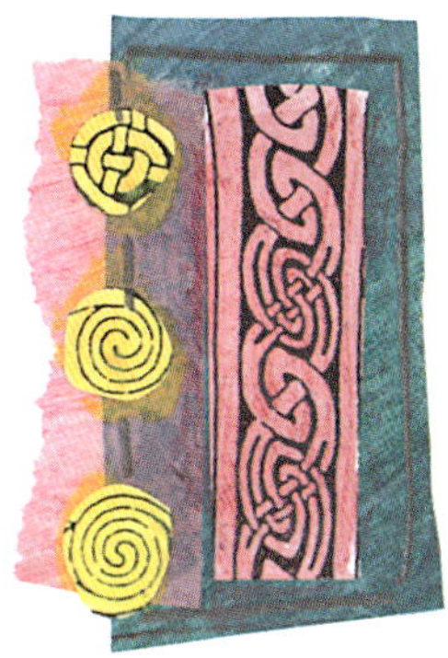

23RD. FERGUS, MAINCHÍN
24TH. ALOYSIUS
25TH. ENAN
26TH. CORMAC, CARTHACH, GARVAN
27TH. FINTAN
28TH. CONALL
29TH. AIDAN, *EITHNE*
30TH. COLMAN, FERGUS
31ST. FAOLAN

ENDA (DIED C.530) FEAST DAY 21ST MAR.

ALTHOUGH ENDA'S ACHIEVEMENTS as one of the leading pioneers of Irish monasticism were real enough, his life is cloaked in legend. In his youth he was a soldier, until his sister – St. Fanchea – urged him to abandon his life of violence. Enda agreed, but only on condition that she gave him one of her nuns as his bride. She did so, but the unfortunate girl fell dead on the eve of the wedding. Enda took this as a sign that he should lay aside his sword and join the Church.

April

1st. Celsus, Aidan
2nd. Conall
3rd. Coman
4th. Ultan, Tierney, Colman
5th. Beacan
7th. Finan, Seanán, Aodh
8th. Ronan, Fáilbhe, Tiernan
9th. Colman
10th. Bercan, Killian
11th. Aodh, Maodhúg
12th. Ernin
14th. Colman, Killian

Cronan of Roscrea (died c.626) f. day 28th Apr.

This name is pronounced *crow-NAWN of ROSS-kray*. Cronan mac Odrain is said to have founded about 50 religious houses, the most famous at Roscrea (Co. Tipperary), which grew into an important monastery. Cronan was renowned for his hospitality, even in old age when he became blind. One legend relates how he transformed water into ale for some weary travellers, making them drunk in the process.

15th. Ruadhán
16th. Ultan, Fáilbhe
17th. Garvan, Aloysius, Eochaidh, Donnan
18th. Eoghan, Laserian
20th. Flann, Enan, Donnan
21st. Bearach
22nd. Callaghan
24th. Dermot
26th. Beacan, Cronan, Donal, Conan
27th. Ultan
28th. Cronan, Suibhne
30th. Ronan, Ciarán

Ronan –
feast days,
8th/30th April

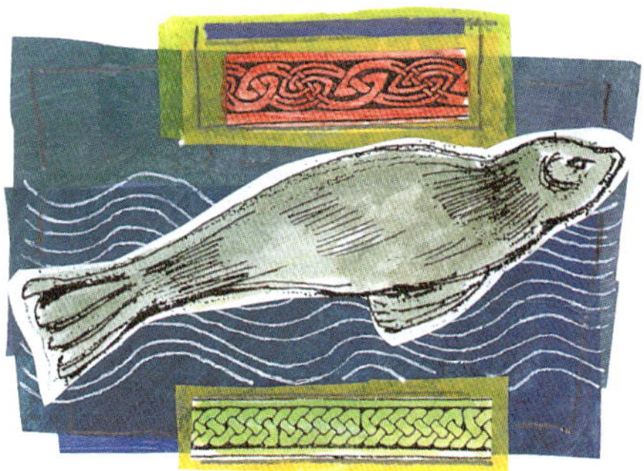

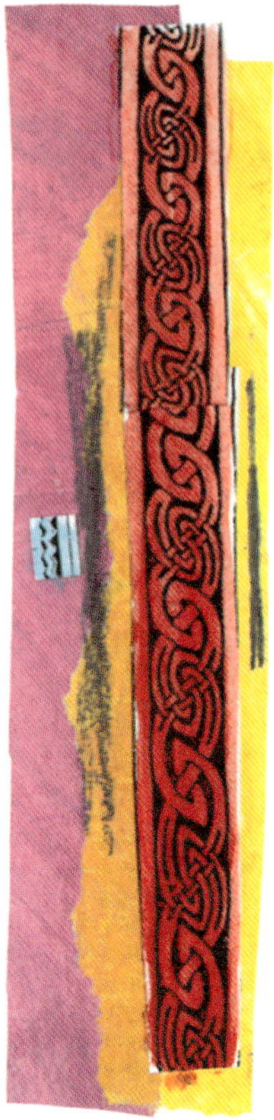

May

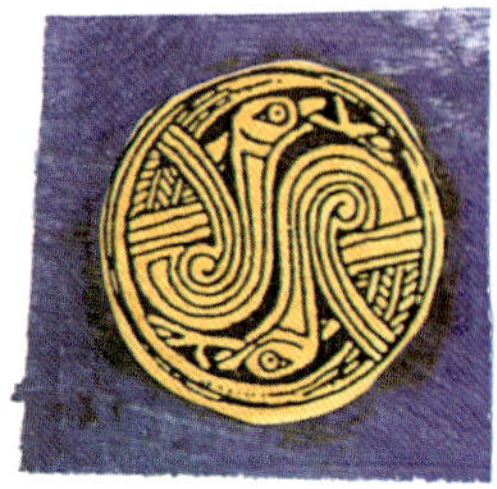

1st.	Ultan, Ronan, Oisin, Mainchín
2nd.	Enan, Colman, Fiachra
3rd.	Cairbre, Conley
4th.	Aodh, Cronan
5th.	Seanán, Faolan
6th.	Colman
7th.	Bercan
8th.	Coman, Odran, Brendan
10th.	Cathal, Aodh, Comhghall

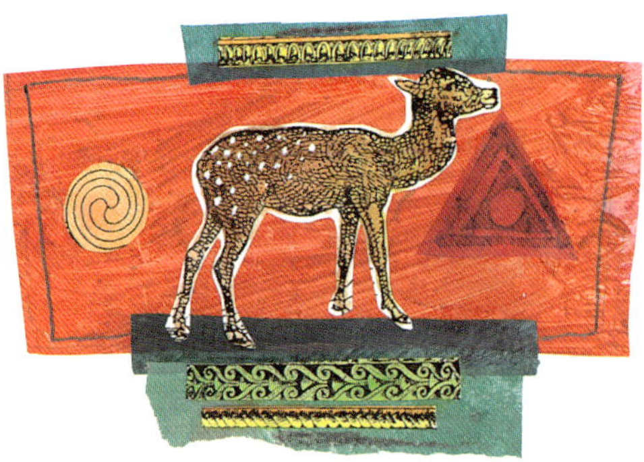

Dymphna – feast day, 15th May

COMHGHALL (c.517–603) FEAST DAY 10TH MAY

THIS NAME (PRONOUNCED *KO-gull*), which means 'fellow-hostage', is sometimes anglicized as Cowal or Cole. Comhghall was born in Ulster and became a pupil of St. Fintan. He lived for a time as a hermit on Lough Erne, where his rule was so strict that seven of his companions died of cold or hunger. In c.555, he established a religious foundation at Bangor, which became the head of a large network of monasteries, numbering more than 3,000 monks. It also served as a base for a series of missionary expeditions to continental Europe.

11TH. KEVIN, FINTAN
12TH. ERNIN
13TH. TIERNEY
14TH. GARVAN, CARTHACH
15TH. COMAN, MUIREADHACH, COLM, *DYMPHNA*
16TH. BRENDAN, ODRAN, ERNAN
17TH. FINNIAN
18TH. BRAN, BREASAL, COLMAN, *AGHNA*
19TH. CUMIN, CIARÁN, *RICHELLA*
20TH. COLMAN
21ST. CUMIN, RONAN, FINBAR, *BRIGID*
22ND. RONAN, CONALL, ALOYSIUS, *AGHNA, LUIGHSEACH*
23RD. CRIOMHTHANN, COMAN
24TH. BERCAN, COLMAN, ULTAN
25TH. DONNCHADH
26TH. COLMAN, BEACAN
27TH. KILLIAN
28TH. EOGHAN, FAOLAN
31ST. ERNIN, EOGHAN

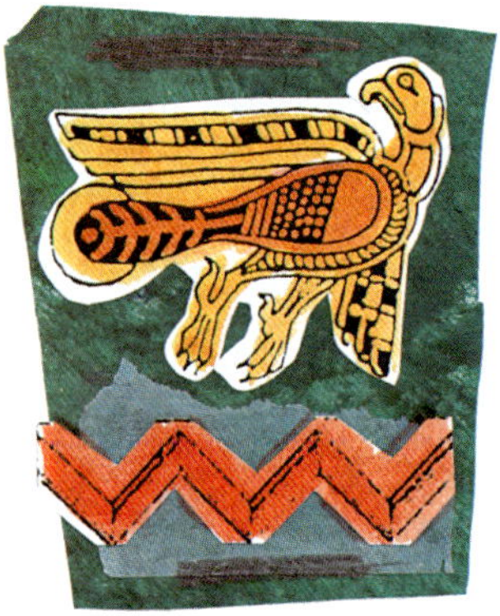

JARLATH (DIED C.550)

FEAST DAY 6TH JUNE

JARLATH (PRONOUNCED *JAR-LATH*), came from a noble family and was noted for his extreme piety – it is said that he performed 300 genuflexions every day – and for his teaching skills. Brendan the Navigator and Colman of Munster were among his pupils. In old age, Jarlath decided to found a monastery where he could end his days. He chose the location after instructing Brendan to take him on a chariot drive. The vehicle broke a wheel at Tuam (Co. Galway) and Jarlath took this as a sign that he had found the ideal spot for his church.

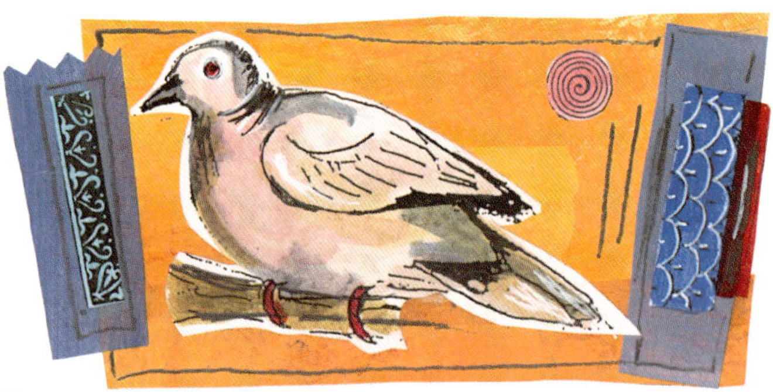

Colm –
feast day, 9th June

1st. Cronan, Colman, Cumin
2nd. Aidan, Seanán
3rd. Kevin
4th. Colm, Ernin, Colman
5th. Bercan
6th. Jarlath, Colman, Faolan, Lonan
7th. Caomhán, Colm
9th. Colm
10th. Bearach
12th. Giolla Chríost, Cronan, Caomhán
13th. Kerill, *Dymphna*
14th. Ciarán
15th. Colman
16th. Sáadna
17th. Aidan, Colman
18th. Colman
19th. Fáilbhe, Caolán
20th. Faolan
21st. Dermot, Suibhne, Cormac
22nd. Cronan, Suibhne
23rd. Faolan
24th. Cormac
26th. Colman
27th. Aodh
28th. Ernin
30th. Fáilbhe, Caolán

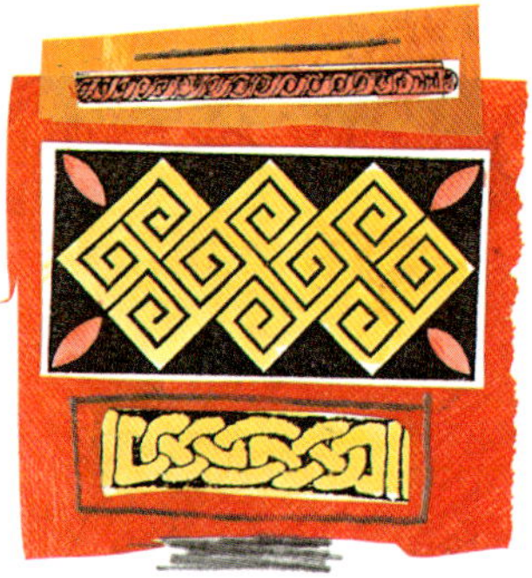

July

1st. Cumin, Ernin, Ultan, Conan

3rd. Killian, Ultan, Maolmhuire

4th. Finbar

5th. Fergus, Ultan, Eadaoin

6th. *Eithne, Blinne*

7th. Tierney, Maelruain

8th. Dermot, Killian, Colman, Tadhg

9th. Garvan

10th. Ultan, Aodh, Cuan, Seanán

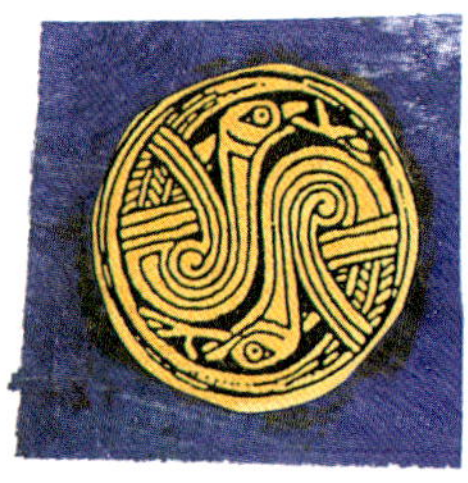

11th. Fáilbhe, Colman, Lonan

12th. Colman, Ultan

13th. Fintan, Ernin

14th. Colman

15th. Ronan, Colman

17th. Flann

18th. Fintan, Cronan, Celsus, Fáilbhe

19th. Oisin, Colman, Ciarán, Aidan, Fergus

20th. Fáilbhe

22rd. Oisin, Colman

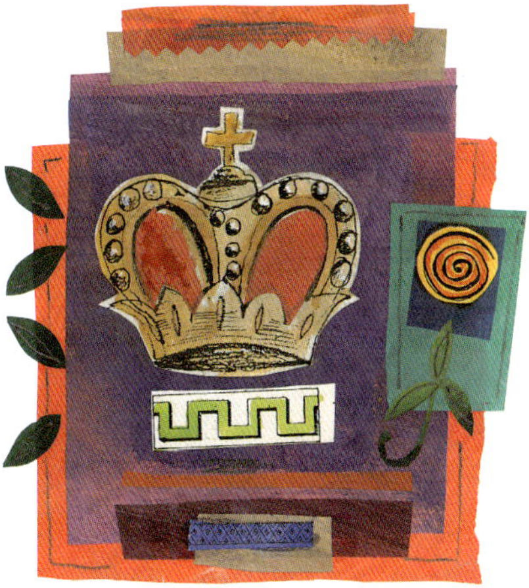

Fergus – feast day, 5th July

24TH. DECLAN, CRONAN, COMHGHALL
25TH. FINBAR, FIACHRA, NESSAN, CAOLÁN, COLMAN
27TH. BRENDAN
28TH. COMHGHALL
29TH. COMAN, CUMIN, CAOLÁN
31ST. COLMAN

MAELRUAIN (D.792) FEAST DAY 7TH JULY

MAELRUAIN (PRONOUNCED *MWALE-RUNE*) was the driving force behind the Culdee movement (from Célé Dé, 'Companions of God'), which spearheaded the reform of the Irish Church in the 8th century. He founded an important monastery at Tallaght (Co. Dublin), where he enforced his austere rule. His personal motto was that there are but 'three profitable things in the day: prayer, labor and study', and that 'labor in piety is the most excellent work of all'. He would probably have been horrified to learn that, in the 19th century, his feast day at Tallaght was celebrated with a boisterous house-to-house procession, accompanied by much dancing and drinking.

August

1st. Colm, Fáilbhe
2nd. Lonan, Fechin, Comhghan
3rd. Aidan, Feidhlimidh, Crohan
4th. Molua
5th. Colman, Ernin, *Ranait*
6th. Aloysius
7th. Cronan, Killian, Aidan, Seanán
8th. Colman

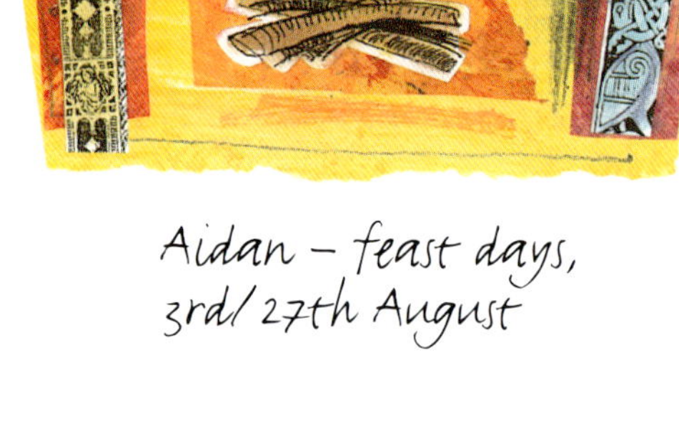

Aidan – feast days, 3rd/27th August

FACHTNA (DIED C.600) FEAST DAY 14TH AUG.

FACHTNA MAC MONGAIGH (pronounced *FOCK-t-na*) was a pupil of St. Finbar and St. Ita. In his youth he was struck blind, but his sight was miraculously restored through the intercession of Ita's sister. In later life, Fachtna went on to found the monastery of Ross Carbery (Co. Cork), becoming its first abbot. This gained great prestige from its monastic school, reputed to be one of the best in Ireland, until it was destroyed by a Viking raid in 991.

9TH. ULTAN, CIARÁN, FEIDHLIMIDH
10TH. CUMIN
11TH. DONNAN, *ATHRACHT*
12TH. LUCAN, IOMHAR, *BRIGID*
13TH. LASERIAN, MUIREADHACH
14TH. FACHTNA, CUMIN, CAOMHÁN
15TH. COLMAN , AODH
16TH. CONAN
17TH. BEACAN, SEANÁN, ERNAN
18TH. ERNIN, COLMAN, ODRAN, RONAN
19TH. ENAN
22ND. CUMIN
23RD. EOGHAN
24TH. FAOLAN
26TH. COMHGHALL, FAOLAN
27TH. AIDAN
28TH. FEIDHLIMIDH
30TH. CRONAN, FIACHRA
31ST. AIDAN, KILLIAN, AODH

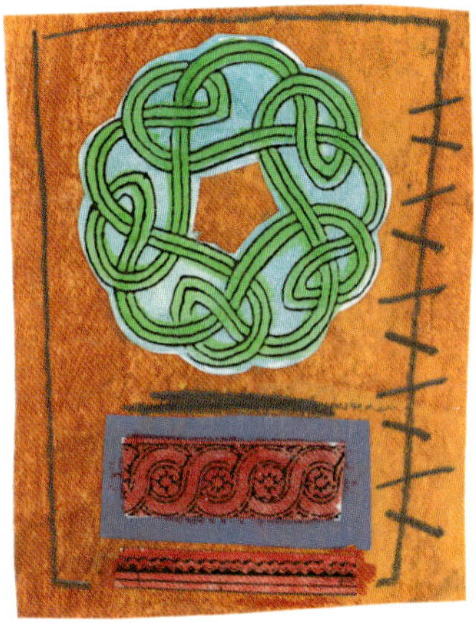

September

1st. Cumin, Fáilbhe
2nd. Colm, Enan, Seanán
3rd. Colman
4th. Ultan, Fiachra, Comhghall, Aidan, Seanán, Cumin
6th. Colm, Colman
7th. Ultan
8th. **Birth of Mary**
Fergus, Fintan
9th. Ciarán, Finbar, Conall
10th. Finbar, Odran, Fergus, Finnian
11th. Colman
12th. Ailbe, Colman
13th. Naomhán
14th. Cormac, Caomhán, *Ailbhe*
15th. **Our Lady of Sorrows**
16th. Laserian, Colman, Seanán
17th. Cumin
19th. Fintan

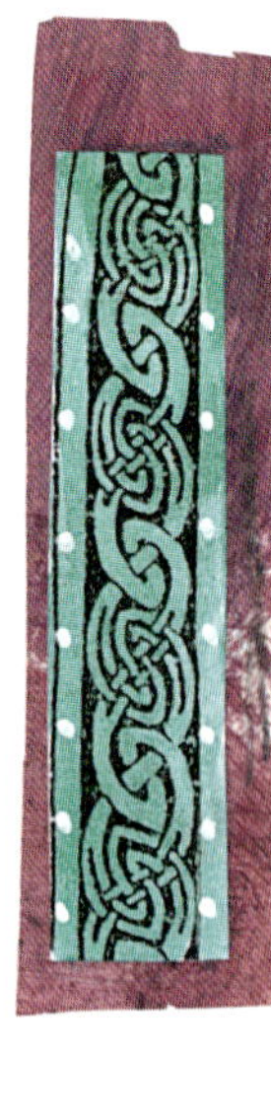

Ultan of Ardbraccan (d.657) feast day 4th Sep.

Ultan is thought to have been one of the first bishops of Ardbraccan (Co. Meath), where there is a well dedicated to him. He was the renowned author of a Life of St. Brigid. Amongst early churchmen, the power of Ultan's hands was proverbial. According to one popular anecdote, he repelled a Viking raid with his left hand, while feeding sick children with his right. This led the chronicler to remark, 'Had it been the right hand that noble Ultan raised against them, no foreigner [Viking] would ever have come into the land of Erin.'

20th. Aidan
22nd. Aodh, Colm, Colman
23rd. Adomnan
24th. Callaghan
25th. Finbar, Colman, Seanán
26th. Colman
27th. Finnian
28th. Dermot, Fiachra
29th. Colm, Ciarán, Nessan, Comhghall
30th. Faolan, Aloysius, *Brigid,* Colman

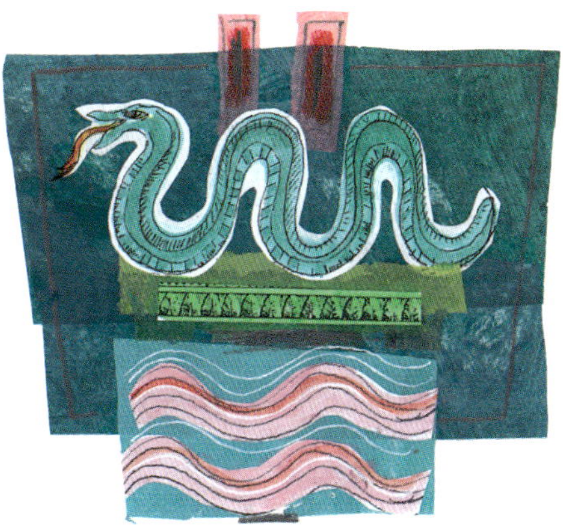

Adomnan – feast day, 23rd September

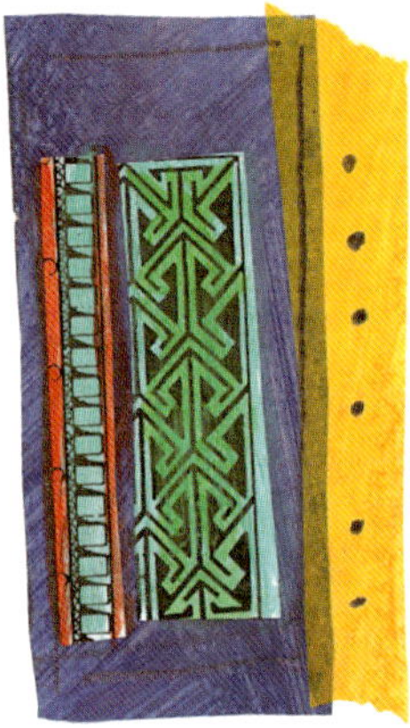

Canice (c.515–99)

feast day 11th Oct.

Canice (or Cainneach) is pronounced *kan-isse*. Canice was born in Co. Derry, the son of a bard. He trained under St. Finnian at Clonard, but moved to Wales to escape an outbreak of the plague. At a later stage, he travelled to Scotland, to accompany St. Columba on a mission to the Picts. In Ireland, he is chiefly associated with the foundation of monasteries at Aghaboe (Co. Laois) and Kilkenny. He also lived as a hermit under a strict rule of silence. On one occasion, he is said to have admonished the birds for singing on the Sabbath.

Kevin – feast day,
16th October

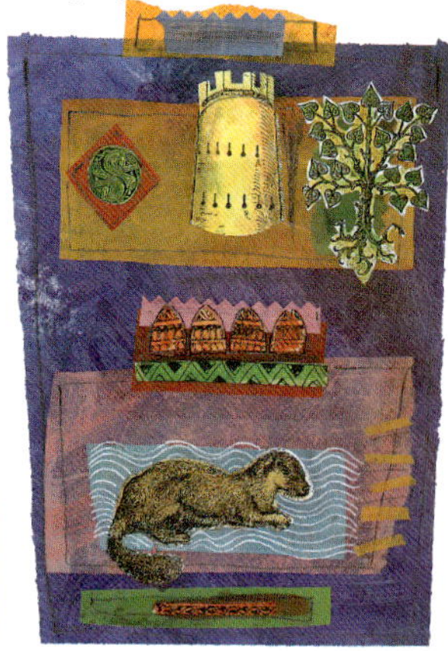

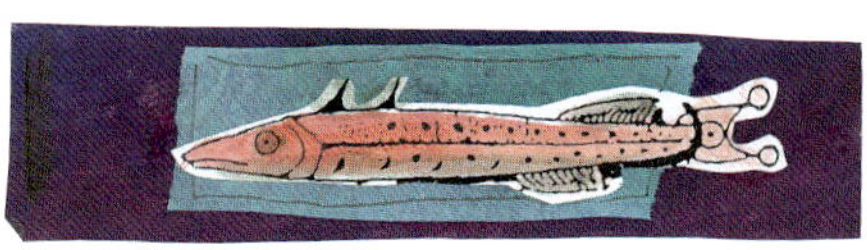

1st. Fintan, Colm, Colman

2nd. Odran

4th. Finan, Colman, Seanán

5th. Baothghalach

6th. Aloysius, Aodh, Colman

7th. Celsus, Comhghall

8th. Ciarán

9th. Aidan, Fintan

10th. Fintan, Seanán

11th. Loman, Canice

12th. Dermot, Fiachra, Aidan, Faolan

13th. Comhghan

14th. Colm

15th. Cuan, Colman, Cormac

16th. Eoghan, Colm, Kevin, Caomhán

18th. Colman

19th. Cronan, Colman, Faolan

20th. Aidan, Fintan

21st. Fintan, Mainchín

22nd. Killian

23rd. Killian

24th. Colman, Lonan

25th. Laserian

26th. Ernan, Odran

27th. Colman, Odran, Ernan

28th. Suibhne, Conan, Colman

29th. Cuan, Aodh, Colman, Caolán

30th. Colman, Feidhlimidh

31th. Faolan, Coman

November

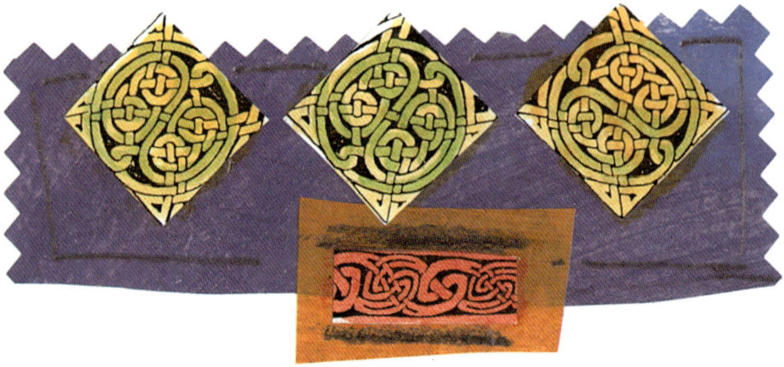

1st. **All Saints' Day**
Cairbre, Lonan, Brendan, Cronan, Aodh
2nd. Aloysius, Aidan, *Caoimhe*
3rd. Caomhán
4th. Tierney
5th. Colman, Faolan, Flannán
6th. **All Saints of Ireland**
Cronan, Aidan
7th. Colman, Fintan
8th. Colm
9th. Beineún, Fintan, *Aodhnait*
10th. Aodh, Coman, Fergus, Ciarán
11th. Cronan, Cairbre, Dubhán
12th. Cumin, Ernin, Lonan, Mainchín
13th. Ernin, *Odharnait*
14th. Lorcan, Colman
16th. Fintan
17th. Aonghus
18th. Ronan, *Hilde*

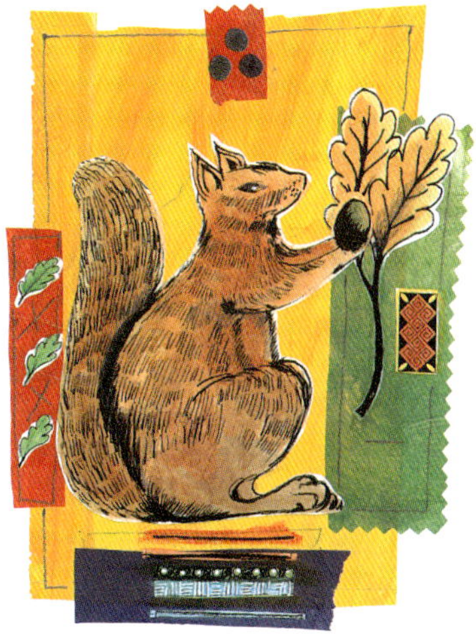

Maeve – feast day, 22nd November

21st. Colman, Garvan, Coman, Aidan
22nd. Ultan, *Maeve*
24th. Bercan, Colman, Cianán
25th. Fergal
27th. Brendan, Cianán, Fianait
30th. Cumin

Cumin the Tall (c.590–c.665) feast day 12th Nov.

Cuimine Fota, better known as Cumin the Tall, was the son of Fiachna, king of West Munster. At an early age, however, he abandoned his princely ways and became a monk. He settled at Clonfert (Co. Galway) where he ran a distinguished monastic school. One of his own hymns is preserved in an early manuscript, The Book of Mulling. At a later stage, he founded a monastery at Kilcummin ('the cell of Cumin'), where there is a well dedicated to him.

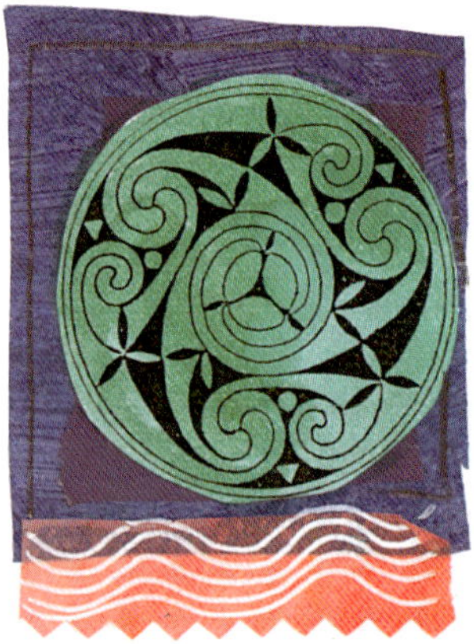

December

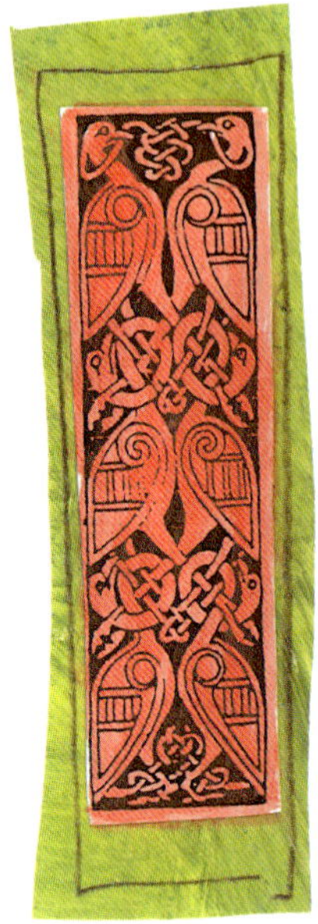

1st. Nessan, Brendan
2nd. Mainchín
3rd. Colman
4th. Bercan, Mainchín
5th. Colman, Seanán
6th. Mellan, Nessan, Beircheart
7th. Colman
8th. Brendan, Finanth

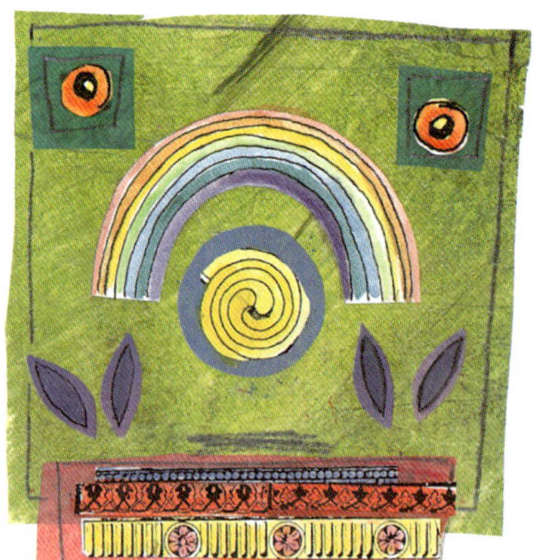

Finnian – feast day, 12th December

FLANNÁN (7TH CENTURY) FEAST DAY 18TH DEC.

FLANNÁN WAS THE son of Turlough, chief of Thomond. According to legend, he went to Rome on a pilgrimage, travelling there miraculously on a floating stone. In Ireland, he is principally associated with Killaloe (Co. Clare). Flannán is said to have founded a monastery there and the present cathedral is dedicated to him. He also appears to have preached in some remote parts of Scotland, as the Flannan Islands near Lewis are named after him.

10TH. COLMAN
11TH. COLM
12TH. FINNIAN, COLMAN
13TH. CORMAC, BRENDAN, COLM
14TH. FINTAN, ERNIN, COLMAN, CORMAC
15TH. FLANN, CRONAN, COLMAN
18TH. CAOMHÁN, FLANNÁN, COLMAN, SEANÁN, EIMHÍN, CUMIN, *RIONA*
20TH. DERMOT, FEIDHLIMIDH, EOGHAN
21ST. FLANN
22ND. ULTAN, EIMHÍN
23RD. COLMAN, RONAN, FEIDHLIMIDH, ERNIN
24TH. CUMIN, SEANÁN, MAOLMHUIRE
25TH. AIDAN
26TH. JARLATH, LASERIAN, COMAN
27TH. FIACHA, COLMAN
28TH. KILLIAN, FECHIN
29TH. MAINCHÍN, ENAN
31ST. ENDA

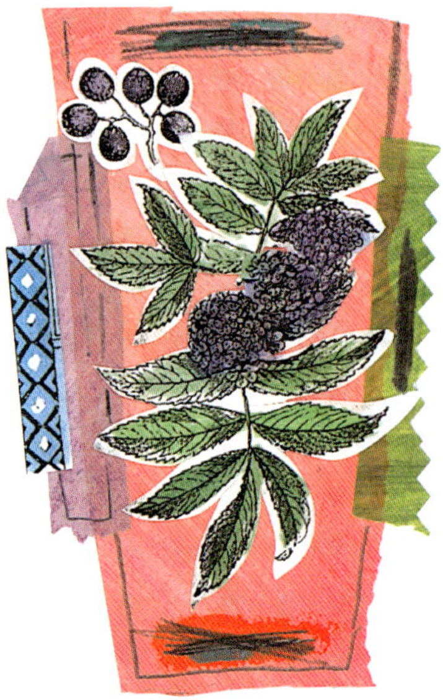